WILLIAMS-SONOMA
COLLECTION

HEALTHY
DESSERTS

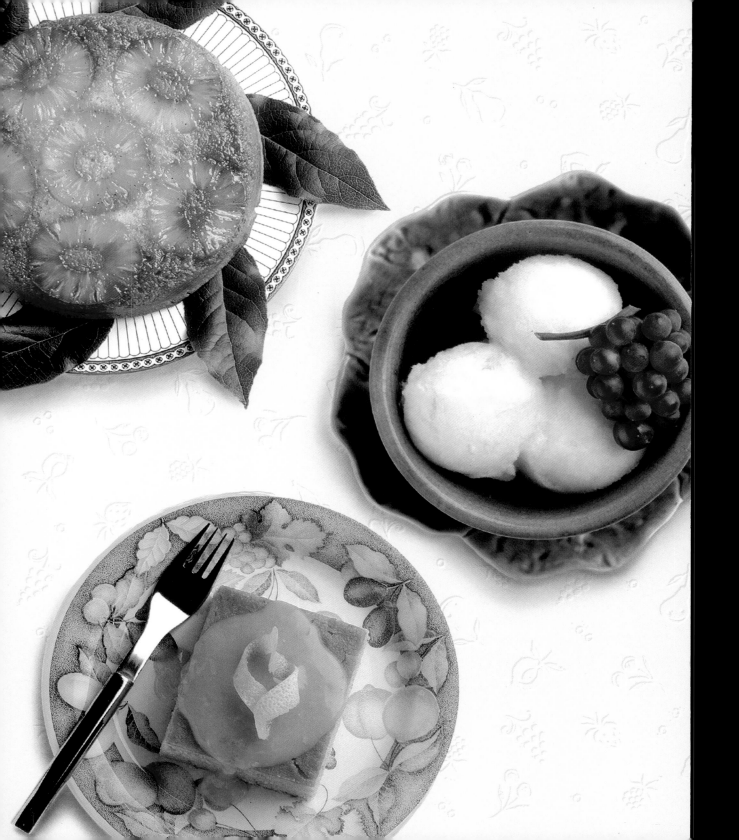

WILLIAMS-SONOMA
COLLECTION

HEALTHY
DESSERTS

GENERAL EDITOR

CHUCK WILLIAMS

RECIPES BY

CYNTHIA HIZER

PHOTOGRAPHY BY

ALLAN ROSENBERG & ALLEN V. LOTT

TIME
LIFE
BOOKS

**Time-Life Books is a division of
Time-Life Incorporated**

President & CEO: John Fahey, Jr.

TIME-LIFE BOOKS

President, Time-Life Books: John D. Hall
Vice President & Publisher: Terry Newell
Director of New Product Development: Regina Hall
Director of Financial Operations: J. Brian Birky
Editorial Director: Donia Ann Steele

WILLIAMS-SONOMA
Founder: Chuck Williams

WELDON OWEN INC.
President: John Owen
Publisher/Vice President: Wendely Harvey
Associate Publisher: Tori Ritchie
Project Coordinator: Jill Fox
Consulting Editor: Norman Kolpas
Recipe Analysis & Nutritional Consultation:
    Hill Nutrition Associates Inc.
    Lynne S. Hill, MS, RD; William A. Hill, MS, RD
Copy Editor: Sharon Silva
Art Director: John Bull
Designer: Patty Hill
Production Director: Stephanie Sherman
Production Editor: Janique Gascoigne
Co-Editions Director: Derek Barton
Co-Editions Production Manager: Tarji Mickelson
Food & Prop Stylist: Heidi Gintner
Associate Food & Prop Stylist: Danielle Di Salvo
Assistant Food Stylist: Nette Scott
Props Courtesy: Sandra Griswold
Indexer: ALTA Indexing Service
Proofreaders: Ken DellaPenta, Desne Border
Illustrator: Diana Reiss-Koncar
Special Thanks: Claire Sanchez, Marguerite Ozburn,
    Jennifer Mullins, Mick Bagnato

The Williams-Sonoma Healthy Collection
conceived & produced by Weldon Owen Inc.
814 Montgomery Street, San Francisco, CA 94133

In collaboration with Williams-Sonoma
100 North Point, San Francisco, CA 94133

Production by Mandarin Offset, Hong Kong
Printed in China

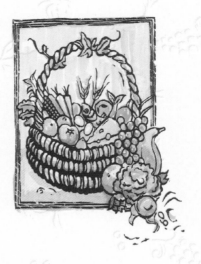

A Weldon Owen Production

Copyright © 1995 Weldon Owen Inc.
All rights reserved, including the right of
reproduction in whole or in part in any form.

Library of Congress
Cataloging-in-Publication Data:

Hizer, Cynthia.
    Healthy desserts / general editor, Chuck Williams ;
recipes by Cynthia Hizer ; photography by Allan Rosenberg
& Allen V. Lott.
        p.   cm. — (Williams-Sonoma collection)
    "A Weldon Owen production"—T.p. verso.
    Includes index.
    ISBN 0-7835-4602-5
    1. Desserts.   2. Nutrition.   3. Low-fat diet—Recipes.
I. Williams, Chuck.   II. Title.   III. Series.
TX773.H573   1995
641.8'6—dc20   95-10208
                                                       CIP

*Cover: The color contrast of bright orange and deep purple provides
plate appeal to Tea-Steamed Apricots & Blackberries (recipe on
page 20). Back Cover: Strawberry & Lemon-Hibiscus Tea Mousse
(recipe on page 103) also uses tea as a nonfat flavoring ingredient.*

HEALTHY DESSERTS

CONTENTS

THE BASICS 6

FRUIT 16

BAKED GOODS 42

FROZEN CONFECTIONS 100

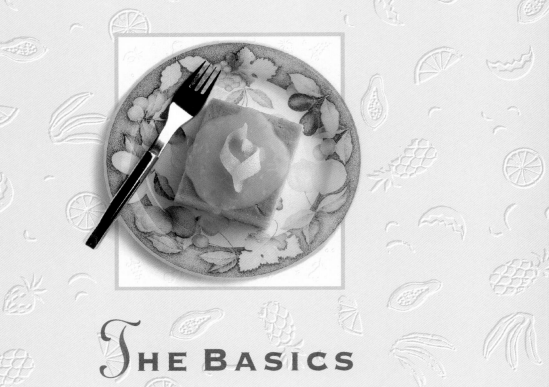

The Basics

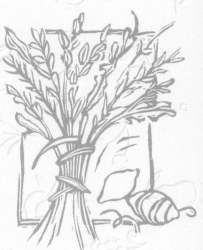

The recipes and nutritional information in this book share the common goal of helping you achieve a balanced diet while continuing to enjoy the traditional pleasure that comes from ending a meal with a special dessert. While this book does not aim to be a weight-loss guide, by making use of its wealth of information and inspiration, you'll most likely find yourself eating in a healthy new way—one that follows today's widely accepted dietary guidelines of 30 percent or fewer calories from fat, about 15 percent from protein and about 55 percent from complex carbohydrates, with more dietary fiber and less cholesterol and added salt. The wide range of ingredients and preparation styles presented in these recipes will also help you achieve another fundamental goal of healthy eating: variety. The following pages explain the many nutritional advantages of the fruit, baked goods and frozen confection recipes that make up *Healthy Desserts.*

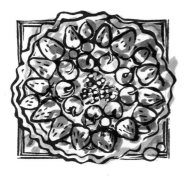

Cooking HEALTHY DESSERTS

It *is* possible to enjoy a dessert that meets all the guidelines of today's healthier approach to eating without giving up all of the joy that comes with a sweet treat. The secrets to cooking such desserts lie in making the right choices of ingredients and in using preparation techniques that do not add unnecessary fat and calories. When choosing ingredients, avoid the traditional cream, butter and eggs that contribute so much fat, particularly saturated fat, and cut down on the sugar that adds so-called "empty" calories to each mouthful.

Fruit, in particular, offers outstanding options for sweets that satisfy and nourish. But even cakes, puddings, ice creams and other dessert favorites can be made in a more health-conscious way, allowing you a full measure of delight. Simple substitutions such as those suggested below, for example, can help you cut some of the fat from desserts and add more nutrients as well. The results may not, at first bite, recall richer counterparts; any change in eating habits, after all, requires some reeducation of the palate. But such desserts will be delicious nonetheless—and they'll be all the more satisfying for the knowledge that you've made them healthier.

MAKING HEALTHY SUBSTITUTIONS

Health-conscious cooks have long taken advantage of a number of simple substitutions to produce delicious desserts that—although somewhat less rich-tasting—are lower in fat, saturated fat, calories and sugar. And in recent years, dairy manufacturers and others in the food industry have made available an increasing number of products to help cooks in their pursuit of healthier desserts. Here are some of the possibilities:

EGG WHITES FOR WHOLE EGGS
All of the fat in eggs resides in the yolks, while the protein- and albumin-rich whites help bind or leaven many desserts. In place of 1 whole egg, try substituting 2 egg whites. When 2 eggs are called for and some of the yolk's richness is required, substitute 2 whites and 1 whole egg.

LOWFAT OR NONFAT YOGURT FOR CREAM OR SOUR CREAM
As lovers of frozen yogurt know, yogurt's creamy consistency and rich, tangy flavor can satisfy like that of far richer cream or sour cream. Although cooking causes them to separate, when no cooking is required, substitute lowfat or nonfat yogurt for cream or sour cream as enrichments or garnishes.

YOGURT CHEESE FOR CREAM CHEESE
Drained of its excess liquid (recipe on page 124), lowfat or nonfat yogurt acquires a thick, spreadable consistency that makes it a good substitute for cream cheese as a spread, garnish or cheesecake ingredient.

BUTTERMILK OR LOWFAT MILK FOR WHOLE MILK
Most dessert recipes calling for whole milk can be made with lower-fat milk instead. Buttermilk, although rich in flavor and consistency, is remarkably low in fat and adds its special tang to baked goods.

WHOLE-WHEAT FLOUR FOR WHITE FLOUR
Ground from the whole grain, whole-wheat flour is higher in fiber, minerals and vitamins than white flour milled from wheat from which the bran and germ have been removed.

Making healthy choices

The choices you make in the food store directly affect your daily and weekly nutritional intake—no less so for desserts than for other courses. Use the following basic information on the two most common categories of dessert ingredients—fruits and dairy products—to help you make wise choices.

Choosing Fruits

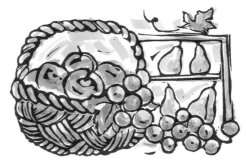

No dessert is healthier than fruit. Virtually free of fat and absolutely free of cholesterol, fruit provides complex carbohydrates and dietary fiber in abundance, as well as such vitamins as A, C and beta-carotene and, depending on the particular fruit, some amounts of essential minerals including calcium, iron and potassium.

Less than a century ago, fruit choices were determined solely by the season. Modern freight methods changed all that, but, unless you feel a pressing need to make a particular recipe that calls for a specific kind of out-of-season fruit, it still makes good sense for several reasons to base your dessert choice on what is in season. Price, of course, is one consideration: What is most abundant is likely to cost less. Quality is another reason: Peak-of-season fruits look and taste their best. Nutrition also matters: Fruits in the best condition deliver the maximum nutritional value. In any season you'll still encounter enough kinds of peak-quality fruit to put together a different dessert whenever you desire.

For best results, wash fruit as soon as possible after purchase. Even fruit with peels that you will discard should be washed so that residue on the peel is not transferred from your hands to the edible portion during peeling.

To ripen stone fruits, place in a paper bag and wait a few days for nature's action. Ripen bananas by hanging the bunches out of direct light. Perhaps the best way to store ripe fruit is right out in the open. A bowl of ready-to-eat fruit on display in the kitchen or dining room provides both seasonal color and a healthy snack alternative.

Although whole-wheat flour is coarser and heavier than white flour, and on its own yields heavier, less fine results, it can be substituted for some of the refined flour in a recipe and still yield good results.

Brown Sugar or Honey for White Sugar

Although sugar in all forms contributes primarily simple carbohydrates and little else to a recipe, less-refined brown sugar does have more than 170 times the amount of potassium in white granulated sugar, more than 85 times the calcium and more than 30 times the iron. Honey, compared to white sugar, has 8 times the calcium, 26 times the potassium and 14 times the iron. Both brown sugar and honey also contribute richer, more wholesome flavors that many health-conscious cooks find appealing.

Cocoa Powder for Chocolate

Produced by extracting cocoa butter from chocolate and then grinding the solid residue, cocoa has significantly less fat than cooking chocolate, yet can impart an intense chocolate flavor to dessert recipes.

Use the list below as a guide to when various fruits are in season and for what to look for when shopping for fruit.

APPLES

In season from late summer to early autumn. Choose firm fruit with good, even color, free of bruises and blemishes; a pronounced aroma is a good sign of ripeness. Refrigerate in plastic.

High in fiber, apples provide generous amounts of vitamins A, B and C, plus iron, potassium and other minerals. One medium apple of any kind contains about 90 calories.

APRICOTS

In season from late spring to late summer. Apricots can be ripened easily at home at room temperature, so buy them fairly firm. Choose unblemished fruit with smooth, velvety skins colored pale yellow to orange. Ripe apricots may be stored in the coldest part of the refrigerator for up to 2 days. Apricots are excellent sources of vitamins A and C, potassium and iron. Three apricots contain about 50 calories.

BERRIES

In season from late spring to mid-summer, depending on variety. Regardless of the type you choose from the many varieties of berries available, select fruit that has good color for its type and is firm, plump and free of bruises, blemishes or mold. Store unwashed in the refrigerator and eat within 1–2 days of purchase. High in vitamin C and other minerals, berries contain less than 40 calories per ½ cup.

CITRUS FRUITS

In season from winter to mid-spring, and available year-round. Whatever type of citrus fruit you buy, seek out fruit with good, bright, even color, free of any soft spots or mold. Store at room temperature up to 1½ weeks or longer in plastic in the coldest part of the refrigerator. All are outstanding sources of vitamin C and provide vitamin A and potassium. An orange contains about 60 calories; a grapefruit, about 74 calories; 1 tablespoon of lemon juice, about 4 calories.

FIGS

In season from late spring to early winter, depending on variety. Select plump-looking, well-shaped figs that feel slightly firm and are free of bruises, splits or flat spots. Refrigerate in a single layer and eat within 2 days of purchase. High in calcium, potassium and niacin, one medium fresh fig has about 40 calories.

GRAPES

Available year-round, depending on variety. Choose plump-looking grapes in full bunches, with good, even, lustrous color for their particular variety. Store in plastic bags in the coldest part of the refrigerator for up to 1 week. A good source of vitamin C, grapes yield on average about 55 calories per ½ cup.

MANGOES

In season from mid-winter to late summer. Seek out mangoes with shiny, unblemished skin that are fairly firm, yielding only slightly to the touch; avoid overly soft, bruised or green fruit. Ripen at warm room temperature; refrigerate when soft and ripe and eat within 1 week. One medium mango provides about 140 calories and offers ample quantities of vitamins A and C as well as calcium, phosphorous and potassium.

PAPAYAS

Available year-round. Choose fruit free of wrinkles or bruises, on which at least half of the green skin has ripened to yellow; continue ripening at room temperature, away from sunlight, until uniformly yellow and soft—3–5 days. When ripe, store in the refrigerator up to 1 week. Extremely high in vitamins C and A, a whole papaya averages about 120 calories.

PEACHES & NECTARINES

In season from late spring to early autumn, depending on variety. Both of these closely related fruits ripen well at room temperature and can be bought on the firm side. Choose those with good, rounded shapes, free of wrinkles, blemishes or any green parts. Ripe fruit will yield slightly to pressure; refrigerate and eat within several days. Both peaches and nectarines provide ample fiber and potassium. Medium-sized nectarines and peaches yield about 65 calories.

PEARS

Available year-round, depending on variety. Avoid any bruised fruit or those that are soft at the stem end or the bottom. Generally sold while still firm and unripe, pears ripen easily at room temperature; when soft to the touch, refrigerate and eat within several days. Pears are very good sources of fiber, calcium and potassium. A medium pear yields about 100 calories.

PINEAPPLES

Available year-round. Pineapples will only ripen on the plant, so purchase only fully ripe fruit. A ripe pineapple should have a pronounced sweet aroma. Avoid bruised or blemished fruit. Refrigerate in plastic and eat within 3 days. Pineapple supplies some vitamin C as well as minerals. One cup yields about 75 calories.

DRIED FRUITS

Intensely flavored and satisfyingly chewy, many forms of sun-dried or kiln-dried fruits play featured or supporting roles in healthy desserts, providing excellent sources of complex carbohydrates, minerals and vitamins. Select recently dried and packaged fruits, which have a softer texture than older ones. Dried fruits contain the same calories as their fresh counterparts, only in more concentrated form. Some of the most popular options include:

APRICOTS The pitted whole or halved fruits are sweet and slightly tangy.

CHERRIES Ripe tart red cherries that have been pitted and dried—usually in a kiln, with a little sugar added to help preserve them—to a consistency and shape resembling that of raisins.

CRANBERRIES Resembling raisins in shape, these have an intense tartness that is often balanced by light sweetening.

CURRANTS Produced from a small variety of grapes, these dried fruits resemble tiny raisins but have a stronger, tarter flavor. If unavailable, substitute raisins.

DATES Although not a dried fruit, the sweet, brown fruit of the date palm tree has a thick, sticky consistency resembling that of candied fruit, and is usually sold with and used like dried fruit.

FIGS A compact form of the succulent black or golden warm-weather fruit, dried figs are distinguished by a slightly crunchy texture derived from their tiny seeds.

PEACHES Halved or quartered, pitted and flattened, dried peaches are sweet and lightly tangy.

PEARS Halved, seeded and flattened, dried pears retain the fresh pear's distinctive profile.

PRUNES A variety of dried plum, with a rich-tasting, dark, fairly moist flesh.

RAISINS From dried grapes, but popular as a snack on their own. For baking, use seedless dark raisins or golden raisins (sultanas).

FREEZING NATURE'S BOUNTY

When fresh fruit is at its peak of season, cooks conscious not only of good health but also a good bargain succumb easily to the temptation to buy in large quantities. This often leads to the inevitable dilemma of what to do with all that fruit.

A century ago, canning was the storage answer. But most cooks now lack the time or the inclination to spend long hours at the stove simmering and sterilizing and today's kitchens for the most part lack the space to store dozens of jars of jams, jellies and sauces.

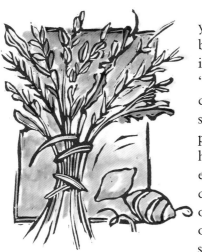

The next time you find yourself buying a bushel instead of a basket, "put up" generous quantities of fresh seasonal fruits simply by using your home freezer. Several kinds of fruit can be frozen without the addition of any sugar or syrup solutions; others require only a simple sprinkling of sugar to ready them for the freezer. All frozen fruit should be used within several months; clearly mark each container's contents and the date of freezing.

BERRIES (EXCEPT STRAWBERRIES)

Gently rinse and drain the berries; spread them in a single layer on a tray, not touching each other. Place in the freezer and, when frozen solid, transfer to plastic freezer bags or containers.

CHERRIES

Rinse the cherries well, then stem and pit them. For every 1 quart (1 liter) of cherries, toss well with ⅔ cup (5 oz/155 g) granulated sugar until the sugar dissolves. Then pack in freezer bags or rigid containers and freeze.

FIGS

Rinse and stem the fruit. Pack in rigid freezer containers and cover with water to which has been added ¾ teaspoon ascorbic acid per quart (liter). Close the containers and freeze.

MANGOES

Peel the mangoes and slice the fruit from the pit, avoiding any fibrous slices. For every 6 cups (36 oz/1.1 kg) of mango slices, add ½ cup (4 oz/125 g) granulated sugar, tossing gently until the sugar dissolves. Pack in plastic freezer bags or containers and freeze.

PINEAPPLE

Peel the pineapple, cutting out all brown eyes; cut out the core and cut into slices or chunks. Pack tightly in rigid freezer containers, close and freeze.

PLUMS

Rinse the plums well, then dry thoroughly. Leave them whole and arrange on a tray in a single layer. Put the tray in the freezer and, when frozen solid, pack the plums in freezer bags.

STRAWBERRIES

Rinse the berries, drain well and hull them. Leave small berries whole and slice larger berries. For every 1 quart (1 liter) of berries, add ⅔ cup (5 oz/155 g) granulated sugar and toss gently until the sugar dissolves. Pack in freezer bags or containers and freeze.

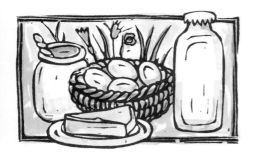

CHOOSING DAIRY PRODUCTS

D airy products, the source of richness and moisture in so many desserts, offer the nutritional benefits of protein, carbohydrates and calcium, but, being animal products, they also carry with them the dietary drawbacks of fat, saturated fat and cholesterol. Fortunately, modern factory techniques for removing fat from milk make it possible to enjoy all of the benefits of dairy products with little or none of the drawbacks. Consider the data below in light of the general recommendations that healthy diets include no more than 300 mg of cholesterol daily and derive no more than 30 percent of calories from fat overall. In an effort to destroy harmful microbes and improve shelf life, most milk products are sold pasteurized. Pasteurizing involves heating to 161°F (80°C) and maintaining that heat for 15 seconds. However, all dairy products are still highly perishable. Make them the last purchase at the store and refrigerate immediately upon return home. Keep open containers covered in the refrigerator to avoid the absorption of other odors. Avoid leaving dairy products in room temperature longer than 30 minutes.

The recipes in this book utilize lowfat and nonfat dairy products whenever possible. Be aware that lessening the fat content may increase the sodium levels in certain dairy products. That happens because when the fat is removed, sodium is needed as a binding agent. For anyone whose healthy

DAIRY PRODUCT

1 CUP (8 FL OZ/250 ML)	CALORIES	FAT (G)	SATURATED FAT (G)	CHOLESTEROL (G)	FAT CALORIES (%)	SODIUM (MG)
Whole Milk	150	8.15	5.07	33	49	120
2% Lowfat Milk	121	4.68	2.92	18	35	122
1% Lowfat Milk	102	2.59	1.61	10	23	122
Nonfat Milk	86	0.44	0.29	4	5	127
Lowfat Buttermilk	99	2.16	1.34	9	20	257
Sour Cream	493	48.20	30.00	102	88	120
Whole Milk Yogurt	139	7.38	4.76	29	48	120
Lowfat Yogurt	144	3.52	2.27	14	22	140
Nonfat Yogurt	127	0.41	0.26	4	3	160

diet needs include a need to limit sodium rather than fat, check the comparatively high amount of sodium in lowfat buttermilk, which has more than twice the sodium of whole milk, and consider an alternative. The sodium levels of all the dairy products are well within the healthy guidelines.

Lowfat milk is available in 1 percent and 2 percent versions. The recipes in this book were tested using 2 percent milk unless otherwise stated. The lowfat buttermilk tested for the recipes in this book contained 1.5 percent fat. Unsalted butter was used in all cases when butter is listed in a recipe.

FINISHING TOUCHES

The way a dessert looks can make a great contribution toward how much satisfaction it brings, especially for children. Use the following garnishing tips, derived from the recipes in this book, as a starting point for adding visual appeal to your desserts—without adding many calories or fat.

CHOCOLATE CURLS & SHAVINGS

Though fairly high in fat, chocolate may be cut into tissue-thin shavings or curls to add interesting visual appeal and a hint of extra flavor to finished desserts. For wide curls, draw a vegetable peeler along the edge of a slightly softened block of chocolate (a handheld hair dryer on the low setting helps). For thin shavings, lightly draw a vegetable peeler across a block of chocolate at cool room temperature.

COCOA POWDER

Free of much of the fat found in the chocolate from which it is extracted, cocoa powder may be dusted over lighter-colored baked goods or iced desserts to add contrasting brown color and a hint of chocolate flavor.

COFFEE

A very light sprinkling of fine, freshly ground coffee, or a scattering of several dark-roasted coffee beans, adds sophistication to iced desserts. A little strong-brewed coffee or espresso may also be poured as a topping over vanilla or chocolate frozen yogurt.

CONFECTIONERS' (ICING) SUGAR

Dusted from a small, fine-meshed sieve over part or all of a dessert's surface, this fine-textured sugar adds a highlight of white color and a hint of sweetness. Be sure to decorate with sugar only just before serving, as it readily absorbs moisture.

EDIBLE FLOWER PETALS

Several common flower species—particularly roses and nasturtiums—have sweet or spicy edible petals that add bright sparks of color and hints of flavor to presentations. Be sure to use only unsprayed, organic flowers purchased especially for eating or homegrown with that use in mind.

FRESH FRUIT

Small, whole berries such as raspberries, blackberries or blueberries may be arranged in decorative patterns or scattered randomly on top of whole desserts or individual servings for a colorful garnish. Thin slices of attractively colored fruit that do not oxidize quickly, such as peaches or nectarines, may also be placed in a fan or other decorative arrangement.

HERBS

Leaves or sprigs of sweet-flavored fresh herbs—most particularly the various varieties of mint—add bright green color and lively, refreshing taste to many desserts.

POMEGRANATE SEEDS

The seeds of the pomegranate look like glistening jewels and add sweet, exotic flavor and crunch when scattered over a finished dessert.

SPICES

Such sweet spices as powdered nutmeg or ground cinnamon may be lightly sprinkled to add extra flavor and a touch of rich brown color. Take care to add them in moderation, so their flavors do not overpower the other ingredients.

ZESTS

The thin outermost peel of citrus fruit adds bright color and literally zesty flavor when cut into shreds or grated as a garnish. (Instructions on page 119.) Very long strips of zest may also be coiled to form attractive flowerlike decorations.

READING A NUTRITIONAL CHART

Each recipe in this book has been analyzed for nutritional composition by a registered dietitian. Beside each recipe, a chart similar to the one below lists the nutrient breakdown per serving. Use these numbers as a tool when putting together meals—and weeks and months of meals—designed for a healthy eating style.

All ingredients listed within each recipe have been included in the nutritional analysis. Exceptions are items added "to taste" and those listed as "optional." When adding salt, bear in mind that you are adding 2,200 mg of sodium for each teaspoon of regular salt and 1,800 mg per teaspoon of coarse kosher or sea salt. Garnishes, substituted ingredients and recipe variations suggested in recipe introductions or shown in photographs have not been included in the analysis.

Quantities are based on a single serving of each recipe.

Protein, one of the basic life-giving nutrients, helps build and repair body tissues and performs other essential functions. One gram of protein contains 4 calories. A healthy diet derives about 15% of daily calories from protein.

Total fat is a measure of the grams of fat present in a serving, with 1 gram of fat equivalent to 9 calories (more than twice the calories in a gram of protein or carbohydrate). Experts recommend that fat intake be limited to a maximum of 30% of total calories.

Cholesterol is present in foods of animal origin. Experts suggest a daily intake of no more than 300 mg. Plant foods contain no cholesterol.

Nutritional Analysis Per Serving:

CALORIES 110
(KILOJOULES 464)
PROTEIN 3 G
CARBOHYDRATES 19 G
TOTAL FAT 2 G
SATURATED FAT 0 G
CHOLESTEROL 0 MG
SODIUM 14 MG
DIETARY FIBER 2 G

Calories (kilojoules) provide a measure of the energy provided by any given food. A calorie equals the heat energy necessary to raise the temperature of 1 kg of water by 1° Celsius. One calorie is equal to 4.2 kilojoules—a term used instead of calories in some countries.

Carbohydrates, classed as either simple (sugars) or complex (starches), are the main source of dietary energy. One gram of carbohydrates contains 4 calories. A healthy diet derives about 55% of calories from carbohydrates, with no more than 10% coming from sugars.

Saturated fat, derived from animal products and some tropical oils, has been found to raise blood cholesterol and should be limited to no more than one third of total fat calories.

Sodium, derived from salt and naturally present in many foods, helps maintain a proper balance of body fluids. Excess intake can lead to high blood pressure or hypertension in sodium-sensitive people. Those not sensitive should limit intake to about 2,400 mg daily.

Fiber in food aids elimination and helps prevent heart disease, intestinal disease and some forms of cancer. A healthy diet should include 20–35 grams of fiber daily.

A Note on Weights and Measures:
All recipes include customary U.S. and metric measurements. Metric conversions are based on a standard developed for these books and have been rounded off. Actual weights may vary. Unless otherwise stated, the recipes were designed for medium-sized fruits.

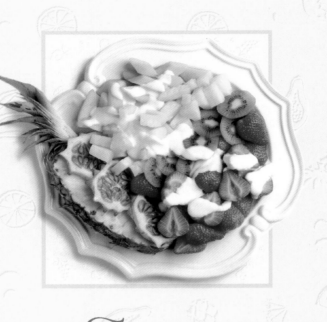

Fruit

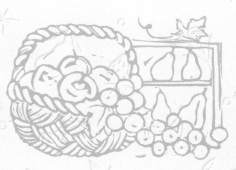

$\mathcal{P}$lucked from tree, vine, or bush, fruit is presented ready for the eating. Historically speaking, it must have been the first dessert, and it remains the purest, simplest and healthiest choice. Simplicity shines through the dessert recipes in this chapter. Some, such as a platter of tropical fruits or fresh raspberries doused with Champagne, require nothing more than slicing or mixing. Others call for only slightly more involved preparation—brief simmering of Asian pears in a spiced syrup, for example, or rapid grilling of colorful pineapple-and-mango skewers. What these desserts have in common is the celebration of the freshness and flavor of seasonal produce. Seasonality is a key consideration when deciding what fruit dessert to make. While modern air shipping makes it possible to get virtually any fruit at any time of year from anywhere in the world, your best bargains and highest quality will always be found in what is in season locally. The wide variety of recipes in this chapter provide myriad delicious options—winter, spring, summer or autumn.

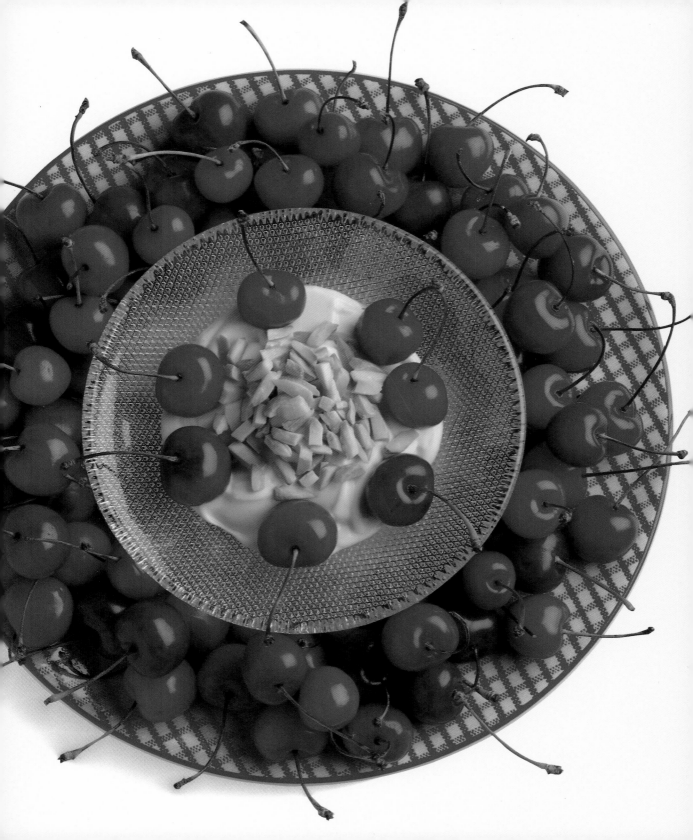

Nonfat dairy sour cream, widely available in food stores, provides a good counterpoint to the intensely sweet cherries. This dish makes a good addition to a dessert buffet, and you can easily assemble it hours ahead of time.

CHERRIES IN ALMOND SOUR CREAM

Serves 6

1½ lb (750 g) cherries, stems
  attached
½ cup (4 fl oz/125 ml) nonfat
  sour cream

1 tablespoon almond extract
  (essence) or amaretto liqueur
2 tablespoons slivered almonds,
  toasted

1. Place the cherries in a shallow serving bowl. In a small bowl, stir together the sour cream and almond extract or amaretto. Sprinkle with the toasted almonds.
2. To serve, set the cherries and sour cream mixture on the table. Let guests serve themselves by dipping the cherries.

*Nutritional Analysis
Per Serving:*

**CALORIES 110
(KILOJOULES 464)
PROTEIN 3 G
CARBOHYDRATES 19 G
TOTAL FAT 2 G
SATURATED FAT 0 G
CHOLESTEROL 0 MG
SODIUM 14 MG
DIETARY FIBER 2 G**

Peak-of-season fruits do well with little embellishment.
A case in point is this Asian-inspired dessert, in which star anise and
scented blackberry leaf tea subtly flavors fresh early-summer fruit.

Tea-Steamed Apricots & Blackberries

Serves 8

8 apricots, 1 lb (500 g) total
weight, peeled and halved, pits
retained
2 star anise, lightly bruised
2 cups (16 fl oz/500 ml) brewed
blackberry tea or plum wine
2 cups (8 oz/250 g) blackberries
fresh mint leaves

1. In a nonreactive saucepan, combine the apricot halves, apricot pits, the star anise and blackberry tea or plum wine.

2. Place the pan over medium heat and bring to a simmer. Cook, uncovered, until the apricots are tender, heated through and fragrant, 3–4 minutes. Remove and discard the apricot pits and star anise.

3. Remove from the heat and add the blackberries. Let stand for 2–5 minutes at room temperature to blend the flavors.

4. To serve, spoon into a serving bowl. Garnish with the mint leaves.

*Nutritional Analysis
Per Serving:*

Calories 41
(Kilojoules 172)
Protein 1 g
Carbohydrates 10 g
Total Fat 0 g
Saturated Fat 0 g
Cholesterol 0 mg
Sodium 1 mg
Dietary Fiber 2 g

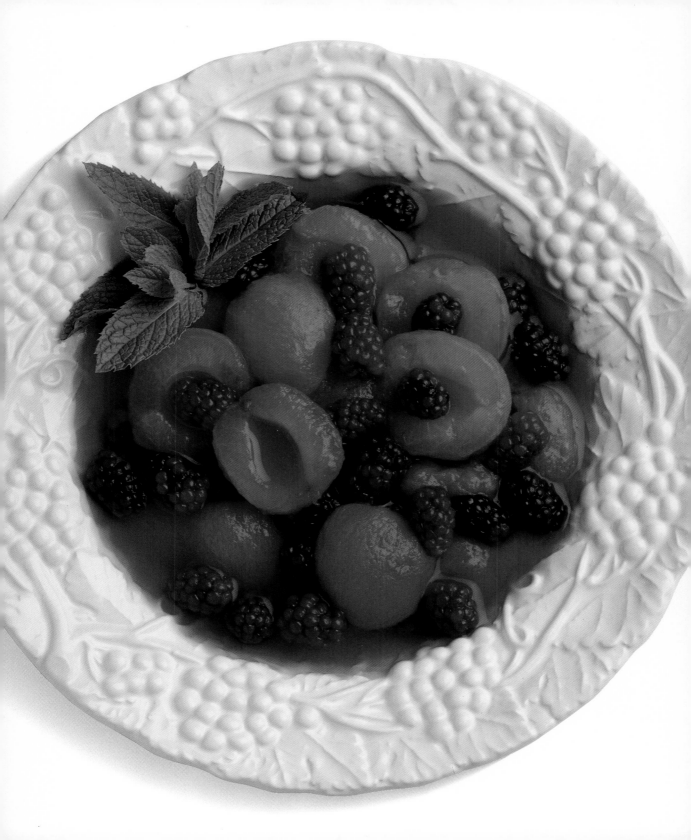

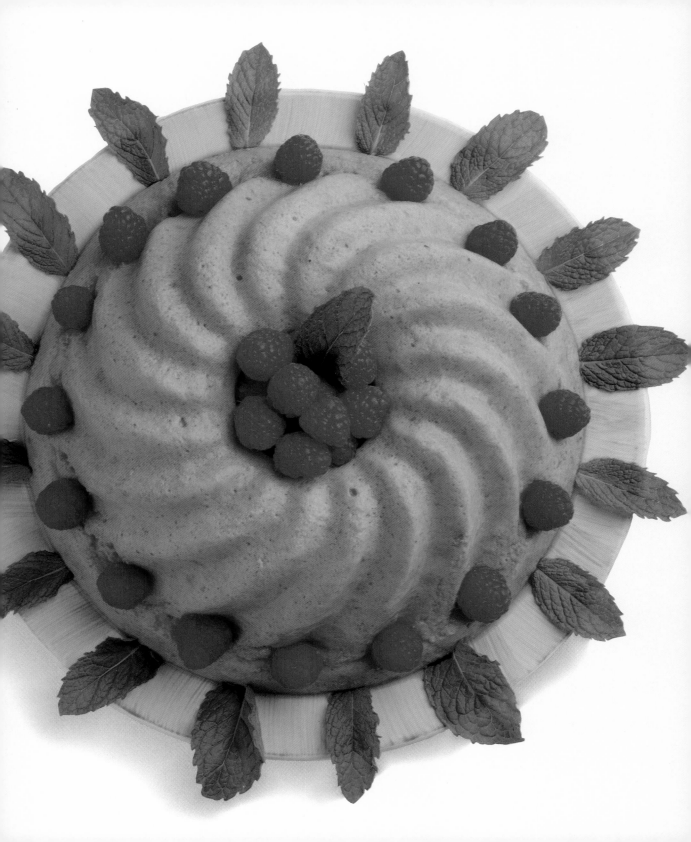

This rich-tasting dessert is a healthy version of a classic French dish. To unmold, fill a baking pan with warm water to a depth of 1 inch (2.5 cm). Set the mold in the water for 10 seconds. Place a serving plate over the top of the mold and invert them. Lift off the mold.

RASPBERRY BAVARIAN CREAM

Serves 16

2 cups (8 oz/250 g) raspberries, plus 24 raspberries

¼ cup (2 fl oz/60 ml) raspberry-flavored liqueur

¼ cup (2 oz/60 g) superfine (caster) sugar

¼ cup (2 fl oz/60 ml) hot water

1 tablespoon unflavored gelatin

3 egg whites, at room temperature

2 cups (16 fl oz/500 ml) Lowfat Crème Anglaise *(recipe on page 127)*, chilled

1 cup (8 fl oz/250 ml) lowfat milk, placed in the freezer for 1 hour

16 fresh mint leaves

1. In a food processor fitted with the metal blade, purée the 2 cups (8 oz/250 g) raspberries until smooth. Pass the purée through a fine-mesh sieve placed over a bowl to remove the seeds. Add the raspberry-flavored liqueur and sugar, stir to mix well and let stand for 10 minutes.

2. Meanwhile, in a heatproof bowl, place the water and sprinkle the gelatin over the top. Let stand for 5 minutes to soften.

3. In a clean bowl, using clean beaters, beat the egg whites until stiff peaks form. Fold together the beaten egg whites, gelatin mixture, raspberry purée and Lowfat Crème Anglaise.

4. In a large chilled bowl, using chilled beaters, whip the milk until soft peaks form. If the milk does not whip easily, return it to the freezer for 15 minutes and then whip again. Gently fold the egg white mixture into the whipped milk.

5. Spoon the mixture into a 2-qt (2-l) pudding mold, angel food, bundt or other tube pan. Cover and refrigerate for at least 4 hours or for up to 24 hours.

6. To serve, unmold onto a serving plate. Garnish with the mint leaves and whole raspberries.

Nutritional Analysis Per Serving:

CALORIES 82
(KILOJOULES 344)
PROTEIN 3 G
CARBOHYDRATES 13 G
TOTAL FAT 1 G
SATURATED FAT 1 G
CHOLESTEROL 17 MG
SODIUM 35 MG
DIETARY FIBER 1 G

Coconut and rum add ample flavor—without added fat and alcohol—to this yogurt sauce topping for the popular tropical fruits listed, as well as the horned melon and pineapple slices used here as a garnish. You can also use the sauce as a dip.

Tropical Fruit Platter

Serves 6

1½ cups (12 oz/375 g) lowfat plain yogurt

½ teaspoon coconut flavoring (essence)

½ teaspoon rum flavoring (essence)

1 pineapple, 4 lb (2 kg), peeled, cored and cut into ½-inch (12-mm) chunks

2 kiwifruits, ½ lb (250 g) total weight, peeled and thinly sliced

2 cups (8 oz/250 g) strawberries, stems removed and berries halved

1 mango, ¾ lb (375 g), peeled, pitted and cut into ½-inch (12-mm) chunks

1. To make the yogurt sauce, in a bowl, stir together the yogurt and coconut and rum flavorings. Cover and refrigerate for 1 hour or up to 2 days.

2. To serve, arrange the pineapple chunks, kiwifruit slices, halved strawberries and mango chunks on a large serving platter. Spoon the yogurt sauce over the fruit.

Nutritional Analysis Per Serving:

Calories 174
(Kilojoules 732)
Protein 4 g
Carbohydrates 38 g
Total Fat 2 g
Saturated Fat 1 g
Cholesterol 3 mg
Sodium 44 mg
Dietary Fiber 4 g

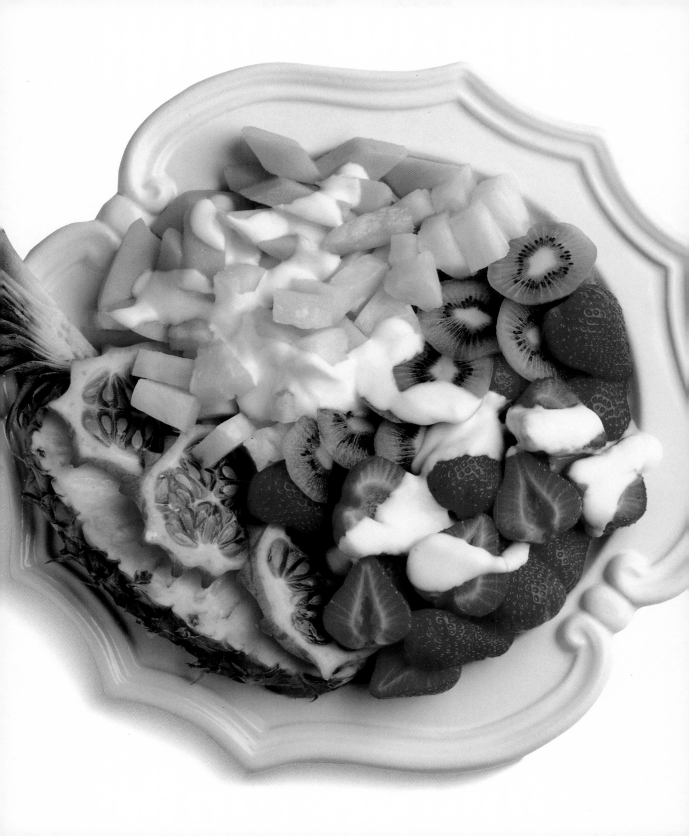

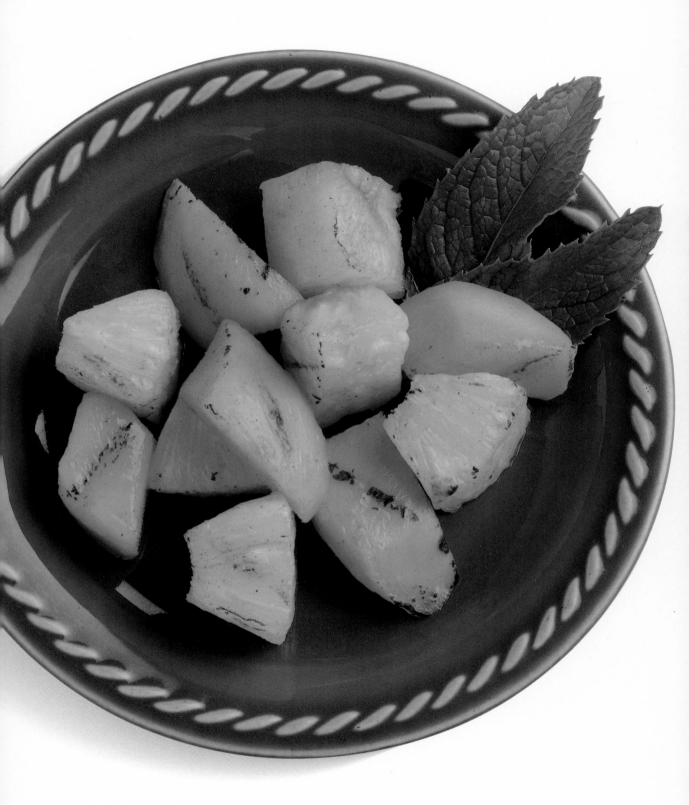

Fresh mangoes, often available in stores when nontropical stone fruits are still ripening on the trees, are rich in vitamin A and beta-carotene. Choose those containing as few fibers as possible, such as the Hayden or Kent varieties.

Mango & Pineapple Kabobs

Serves 6

2 ripe mangoes, 1½ lb (750 g) total weight

1 pineapple, 4 lb (2 kg), peeled, cored and cut into 1-inch (2.5-cm) cubes

½ cup (4 fl oz/125 ml) fresh lime juice

½ teaspoon ground cinnamon

1. Prepare a fire in a charcoal grill or preheat a broiler (griller). If using wooden or bamboo skewers, soak in a container with water to cover for 30 minutes to prevent burning.

2. To prepare each mango, using a sharp paring knife, cut it in half lengthwise, circling the flat seed, and twist the halves apart. Remove and discard the seed. Cradle a mango half in your hand and, using the paring knife, carefully score the pulp in 1-inch (2.5-cm) diamonds, then cut along the base of each diamond to release it.

3. If you have soaked the skewers, drain them. Alternate the mango diamonds and pineapple cubes on 6 skewers and place them on a platter. Drizzle the fruits with the lime juice and sprinkle with the cinnamon.

4. Place the kabobs on the grill rack or broiler rack and cook, turning frequently, until the fruit is heated through, sizzling and crispy, 5–10 minutes. Watch carefully that the fruit does not overcook and begin to fall from the skewers.

5. To serve, slide the fruit from the skewers and place on individual plates.

Nutritional Analysis Per Serving:

Calories 134 (Kilojoules 564)
Protein 1 g
Carbohydrates 35 g
Total Fat 1 g
Saturated Fat 0 g
Cholesterol 0 mg
Sodium 3 mg
Dietary Fiber 3 g

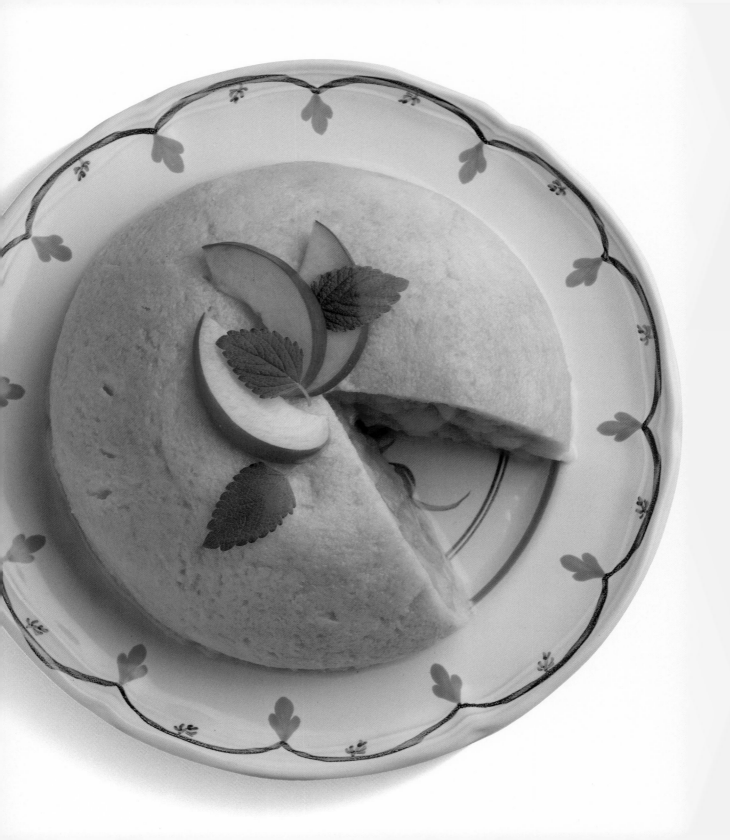

Although raspberries are most often used for summer puddings, nectarines bring their own bright flavor and color to this classic English dessert. Use only fully ripe fruit to get enough juice to hold the pudding together. A deep mixing bowl may replace the pudding mold.

Summer Pudding

Serves 6

2½ lb (1.25 kg) very ripe nectarines, peeled, pitted and cut into ½-inch (12-mm) cubes, juice retained

½ cup (4 oz / 125 g) Vanilla Sugar *(recipe on page 125)* or granulated sugar

½ lb (250 g) firm white bread, thinly sliced and crust removed

2 tablespoons crystallized ginger, finely chopped

1. In a large mixing bowl, combine the nectarines, accumulated juices and Vanilla Sugar or granulated sugar. Stir to mix well. Let the mixture stand at room temperature for 30 minutes.

2. Meanwhile, line the bottom and sides of a 1½-qt (1.5-l) pudding mold with a single layer of the bread slices, trimming them so they fit snugly. Trim additional slices as needed to cover the top and set aside.

3. Pour off the accumulated fruit juice into a separate shallow bowl, leaving the fruit dense and almost dry. Stir the crystallized ginger into the nectarines.

4. Remove the bread slices lining the bowl one by one, dip each one into the juice and then fit it back into the bowl. Fill any holes with small leftover pieces of bread. Spoon the fruit into the bowl; it should almost reach the top. Then dip the bread pieces reserved for the top in the juice and place over the fruit. Cover with the remaining fruit juice.

5. Place a heavy plate or other heavy, flat object that fits just inside the rim of the bowl on top. Refrigerate overnight.

6. To serve, unmold (instructions on page 23). Cut the pudding into wedges and place on individual plates.

Nutritional Analysis Per Serving:

Calories 267 (Kilojoules 1,122)
Protein 4 g
Carbohydrates 61 g
Total Fat 2 g
Saturated Fat 0 g
Cholesterol 0 mg
Sodium 187 mg
Dietary Fiber 4 g

Also known as pear apples and nashi fruits, Asian pears have the size,
shape and some of the crispness of apples. You could substitute a soft variety
of apple, such as a Jonathan, in this light, refreshing dessert.

Asian Pear Compote

Serves 4

1 cup (8 oz/250 g) sugar
2 star anise, bruised
½ cup (4 fl oz/125 ml) water
grated zest and juice of 1 lemon
4 large Asian pears, 2 lb (1 kg)
    total weight, peeled, cut into
    quarters, cored and cut into
    ½-inch (12-mm) cubes

1. In a large saucepan, combine the sugar, star anise
and water. Bring to a boil over medium heat, stirring
to dissolve the sugar. Reduce the heat to low and
simmer, uncovered, until the steam is fragrant, about
5 minutes.
2. Add the lemon zest and juice and pears. Simmer,
uncovered, stirring occasionally, until the pears are
translucent and liquid has reduced to a syrup, about
10 minutes. Remove and discard the star anise.
3. To serve, spoon into individual bowls.

*Nutritional Analysis
Per Serving:*

**CALORIES 332
(KILOJOULES 1,395)
PROTEIN 0 G
CARBOHYDRATES 86 G
TOTAL FAT 1 G
SATURATED FAT 0 G
CHOLESTEROL 0 MG
SODIUM 1 MG
DIETARY FIBER 4 G**

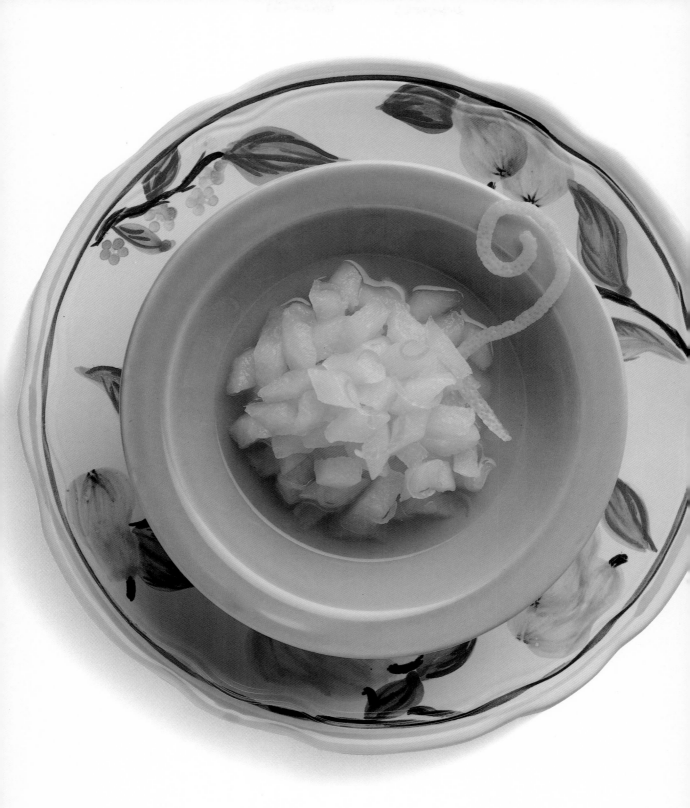

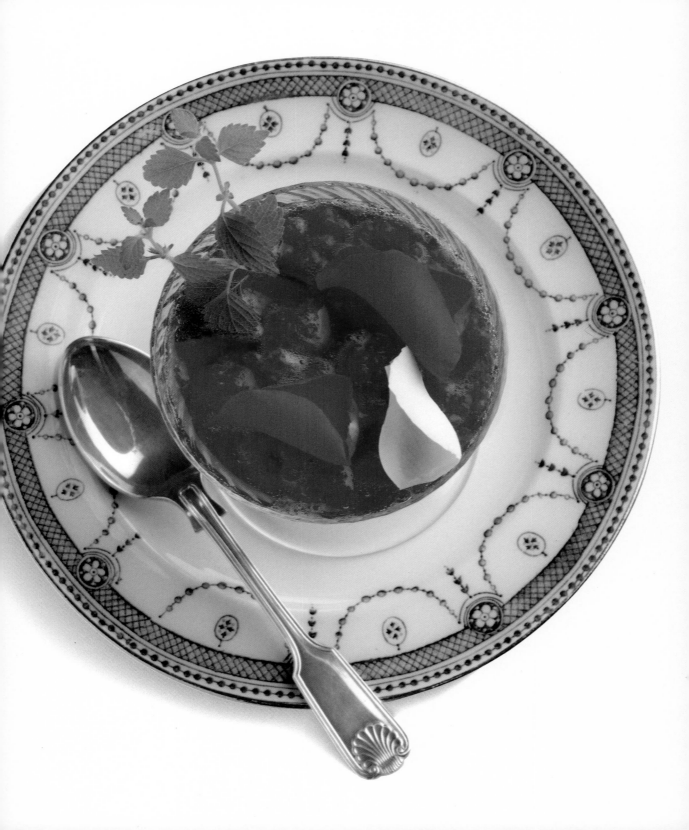

Think of this as an elegant chilled fruit soup for summer. You have the option of making it with or without alcohol. You can also substitute unsweetened frozen raspberries, but some of the fresh fruit's texture will be lost.

CHAMPAGNE RASPBERRIES

Serves 6

3 cups (12 oz/375 g) fresh
   raspberries
2 tablespoons framboise or
   rose water

2 cups (16 fl oz/500 ml)
   Champagne or other sparkling
   wine or sparkling water
fresh mint leaves
pesticide-free rose petals, optional

1. In a bowl, using the back of a large spoon, lightly crush the berries to release their juices and fragrance. Sprinkle the liqueur or rose water over the berries and let stand for 10 minutes.
2. To serve, spoon the raspberries and their juices into individual bowls. Pour an equal amount of the Champagne or sparkling water into each bowl. Garnish with the mint leaves and the rose petals, if using.

*Nutritional Analysis
Per Serving:*

**CALORIES 95
(KILOJOULES 400)
PROTEIN 1 G
CARBOHYDRATES 9 G
TOTAL FAT 0 G
SATURATED FAT 0 G
CHOLESTEROL 0 MG
SODIUM 4 MG
DIETARY FIBER 3 G**

Use any sweet variety of seedless grapes for a quick preparation or delicious seeded grapes, if you don't mind the extra work of getting out the seeds. The grapes will keep in the refrigerator for up to 10 days.

SPIKED RED GRAPES

Serves 6

1 lb (500 g) seedless red grapes, stemmed

½ cup (4 fl oz/125 ml) raspberry vinegar

1 tablespoon balsamic vinegar

½ cup (4 fl oz/125 ml) rosé wine or sparkling water

¾ cup (6 oz/185 g) sugar

4 whole cloves, lightly bruised

1 cinnamon stick, 3 inches (7.5 cm) long

6 cardamom seeds, lightly crushed

1. Place the grapes in a 2-qt (2-l) glass jar or other glass or ceramic container.

2. In a saucepan over medium heat, combine the raspberry and balsamic vinegars, wine or sparkling water, sugar, cloves, cinnamon stick and cardamom seeds. Heat, stirring occasionally, until the sugar dissolves, about 5 minutes. Remove from the heat and let cool slightly.

3. Pour the vinegar mixture over the grapes. Cover the container tightly and refrigerate for at least 2 days and for up to 10 days, inverting the container occasionally to make sure they are marinating evenly.

4. To serve, remove and discard the cloves, cinnamon stick and cardamom seeds before spooning into individual bowls.

Nutritional Analysis
Per Serving:

CALORIES 175
(KILOJOULES 737)
PROTEIN 1 G
CARBOHYDRATES 43 G
TOTAL FAT 0 G
SATURATED FAT 0 G
CHOLESTEROL 0 MG
SODIUM 3 MG
DIETARY FIBER 0 G

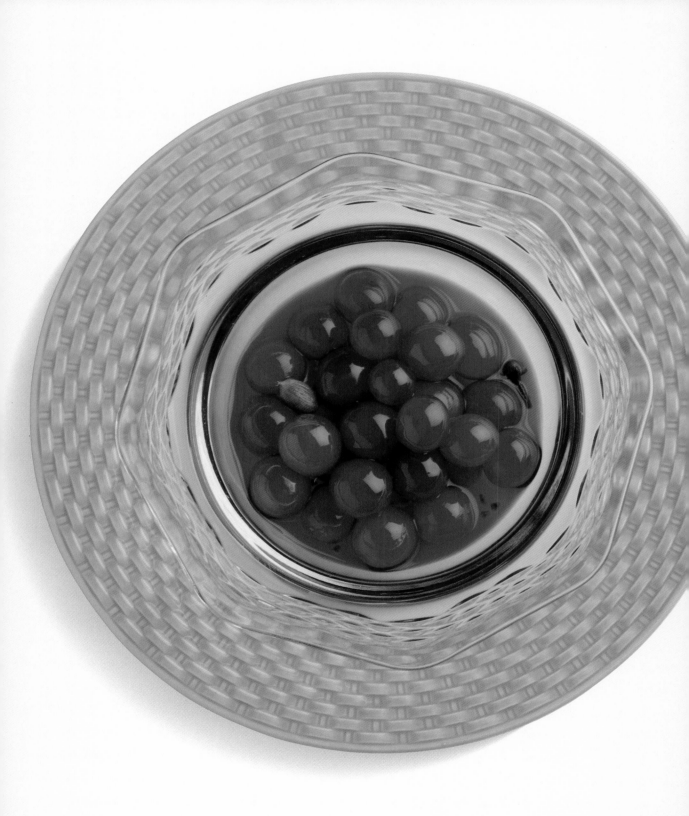

A crumb crust made from chocolate cookies makes this a "no-bake" pie that tastes great. The filling of Lowfat Crème Anglaise, a classic custard sauce, should be made thick enough to spoon rather than pour.

STRAWBERRY TART

Serves 8

20 chocolate wafer cookies, crumbled

3 tablespoons vegetable oil

1 cup (8 fl oz/250 ml) Lowfat Crème Anglaise made with ¼ cup (1 oz/30 g) cornstarch (cornflour) *(recipe on page 127)*

1 tablespoon firmly packed light brown sugar

3 cups (12 oz/375 g) strawberries, stems removed and sliced

2 tablespoons apricot fruit spread

1. In a food processor fitted with the metal blade, combine the cookies and vegetable oil and process to chop finely, 10–15 seconds. Pat the crumb mixture into the bottom of a 9-inch (23-cm) pie pan. Refrigerate to set the crust, about 15 minutes.

2. In a bowl, stir together the Lowfat Crème Anglaise and brown sugar. Spoon it onto the prepared pie crust, smoothing it with a spatula. Refrigerate to set the filling, about 15 minutes.

3. Arrange the sliced strawberries on top of the tart filling. In a small saucepan over low heat, melt the fruit spread until it liquefies, about 1 minute. Brush the warmed spread in a thin layer over the strawberries. Refrigerate to set the glaze, about 15 minutes.

4. To serve, cut into wedges and place on plates.

Nutritional Analysis Per Serving:

CALORIES 180
(KILOJOULES 754)
PROTEIN 2 G
CARBOHYDRATES 25 G
TOTAL FAT 8 G
SATURATED FAT 2 G
CHOLESTEROL 16 MG
SODIUM 104 MG
DIETARY FIBER 1 G

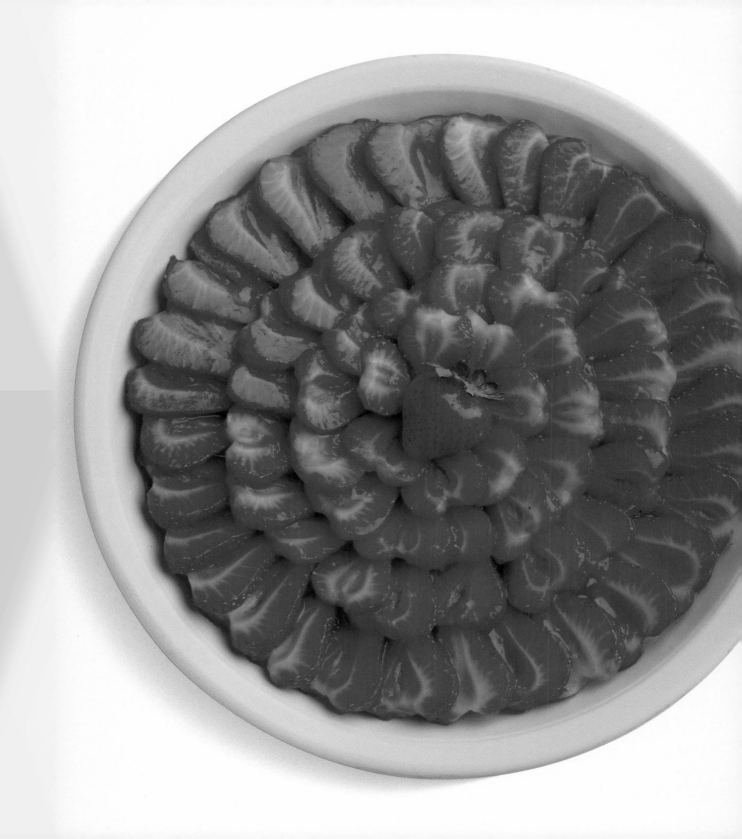

Prune plums, also known as French prune plums or Italian plums, come into season just as other stone fruits finish. Commonly destined to be dried as prunes, they are full of sugar and delicious fresh in this robust taste of fall.

Autumn Pudding

Serves 6

3 cups (18 oz/560 g), about 1½ lb (750 g), diced ripe prune plums

3 cups (12 oz/375 g) ripe blackberries

2 tablespoons juniper berries in a cheesecloth sack

½ cup (4 oz/125 g) sugar

6 thick slices day-old, firm white bread, crusts removed and bread crumbled (3 cups/6 oz/185 g)

½ cup (4 oz/125 g) lowfat plain yogurt

1 teaspoon fresh lemon juice

1. In a saucepan over medium-low heat, combine the plums, blackberries, juniper berries and sugar. Cook, stirring occasionally, until the fruits swell, 10 minutes. Using the back of a large spoon, lightly crush the fruits to release their juices, then remove from the heat and let cool to room temperature. Remove and discard the juniper berries.

2. Beginning with the bread, alternate layers of the crumbled bread and the cooled fruits in large goblets until everything is used. Pour any remaining fruit juice over the top. Cover and chill for several hours.

3. In a small bowl, stir together the yogurt and lemon juice.

4. To serve, top each serving with an equal amount of the yogurt mixture.

Nutritional Analysis Per Serving:

Calories 263
(Kilojoules 1,104)
Protein 4 g
Carbohydrates 61 g
Total Fat 2 g
Saturated Fat 0 g
Cholesterol 1 mg
Sodium 152 mg
Dietary Fiber 3 g

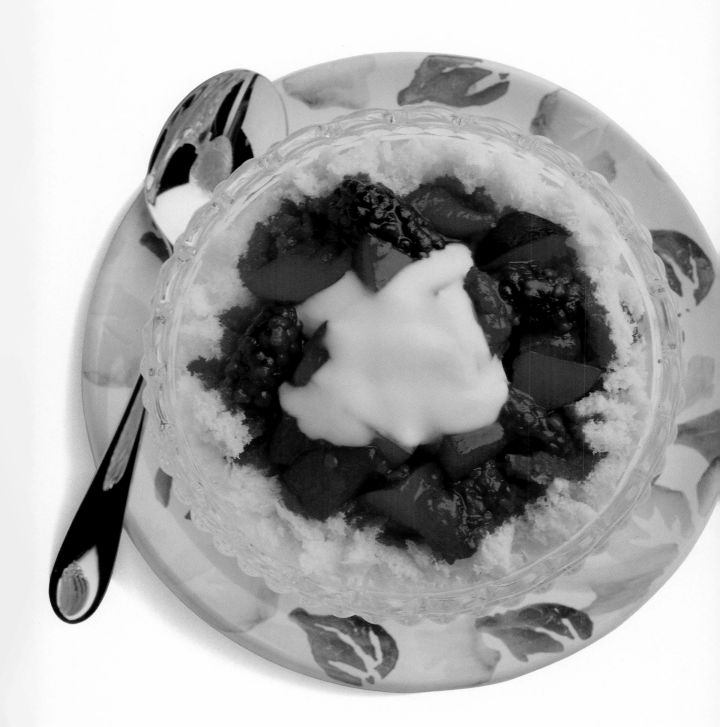

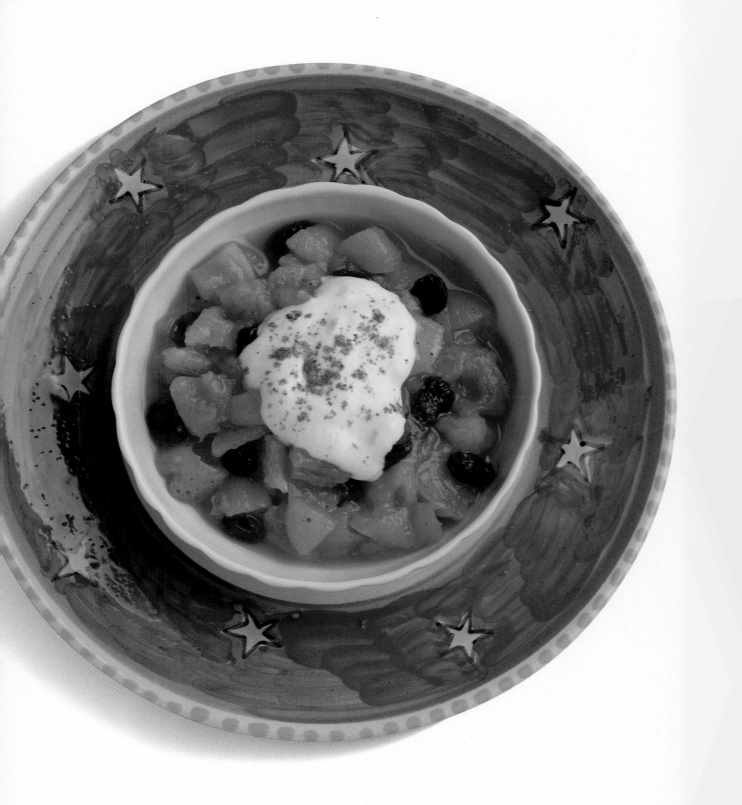

Recalling a time before modern air freight, when the only fruits widely available in winter were likely to be dried, this slowly baked dessert is good served warm on its own or alongside angel food cake or rice pudding.

WINTER FRUIT COMPOTE

Serves 4

2 tablespoons crystallized ginger, finely chopped

2 tablespoons honey, Vanilla Sugar *(recipe on page 125),* or granulated sugar

¼ teaspoon freshly grated nutmeg, plus freshly grated nutmeg

½ cup (4 fl oz/125 ml) water

½ cup (4 fl oz/125 ml) apple juice or port wine

2 pears, 10 oz (315 g) total weight, peeled, cored and chopped

½ cup (3 oz/90 g) dried apricots, chopped

½ cup (3 oz/90 g) dried pears or peaches, chopped

¼ cup (1½ oz/45 g) raisins

½ cup (4 oz/125 g) Yogurt Cheese *(recipe on page 124),* at room temperature

1. Preheat an oven to 350°F (180°C).

2. In a flameproof baking dish, combine the ginger, honey or Vanilla Sugar or granulated sugar, the ¼ teaspoon of the nutmeg, water, apple juice or port, fresh pears, dried apricots and dried pears or peaches. Place over medium-high heat and bring to a boil. Remove from the heat and let stand for 10 minutes to allow fruits to steep in the juices.

3. Bake, uncovered, until the fruit is tender and translucent, 20–30 minutes. Remove from the oven, stir in the raisins and return to the oven for 10 minutes longer.

4. To serve, spoon into individual bowls and top each serving with an equal amount of the Yogurt Cheese. Garnish with the remaining grated nutmeg.

Nutritional Analysis Per Serving:

**CALORIES 291
(KILOJOULES 1,222)
PROTEIN 5 G
CARBOHYDRATES 71 G
TOTAL FAT 1 G
SATURATED FAT 0 G
CHOLESTEROL 1 MG
SODIUM 29 MG
DIETARY FIBER 4 G**

Baked Goods

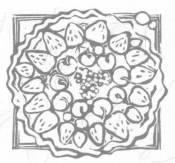

A heavenly angel food cake flavored with cocoa, autumn pears nestled in a pastry shell and spiced with cinnamon and ginger, a homespun cobbler of summer fruit covered with a biscuit topping, and crisp licorice-scented Italian biscotti with whole aniseeds are undeniably satisfying baked desserts. Nutritionists explain the popularity of baked goods by pointing to their high percentage of grains, the rich sources of the complex carbohydrates that do such a good job of pacifying the appetite, and testify that home-made goods are free of the preservatives and additives found in some commercial products. But those whose souls are stirred by baked desserts might prefer the explanation that, with every taste, they return us to the kitchens of childhood, where wonderful things came out of the oven. While the desserts in this chapter employ principles of healthy eating, the fact remains that with one scent, look and bite, baked desserts are wonderfully reminiscent of the traditional foods of days gone by.

These dense, lowfat brownies should satisfy even serious chocolate addicts, who might never suspect that the rich texture comes from puréed prunes. If canned prunes are unavailable, simmer dried prunes in water to cover for 15 minutes before puréeing.

Cocoa Brownies

Makes 12 brownies

½ cup (3 oz/90 g) canned, drained pitted prunes, puréed
½ cup (4 fl oz/125 ml) water, boiling
3 large egg whites, lightly beaten
2 tablespoons vegetable oil or walnut oil

1 cup (8 oz/250 g) Vanilla Sugar *(recipe on page 125)* or granulated sugar
⅓ cup (1 oz/30 g) unsweetened cocoa
1 cup (5 oz/155 g) all-purpose (plain) flour
1 teaspoon baking powder
½ teaspoon salt
¼ cup (1 oz/30 g) chopped walnuts

1. Preheat an oven to 350°F (180°C). Coat an 8-inch (20-cm) square baking pan with nonstick cooking spray.
2. In a large bowl, combine the prune purée, water, egg whites, vegetable or walnut oil and Vanilla Sugar or granulated sugar. Using a wooden spoon, beat until thoroughly blended.
3. In a medium bowl, stir together the cocoa, flour, baking powder and salt. Add the flour mixture to the prune mixture. Stir to mix well.
4. Spoon the batter into the prepared pan. Sprinkle the walnuts evenly over the top. Bake until the top springs back when touched, about 30 minutes. Transfer to a rack to cool completely in the pan, about 30 minutes.
5. To serve, cut into squares. Store in a tightly covered container for several days.

Nutritional Analysis Per Brownie:

**Calories 179
(Kilojoules 752)
Protein 3 g
Carbohydrates 34 g
Total Fat 4 g
Saturated Fat 1 g
Cholesterol 0 mg
Sodium 147 mg
Dietary Fiber 2 g**

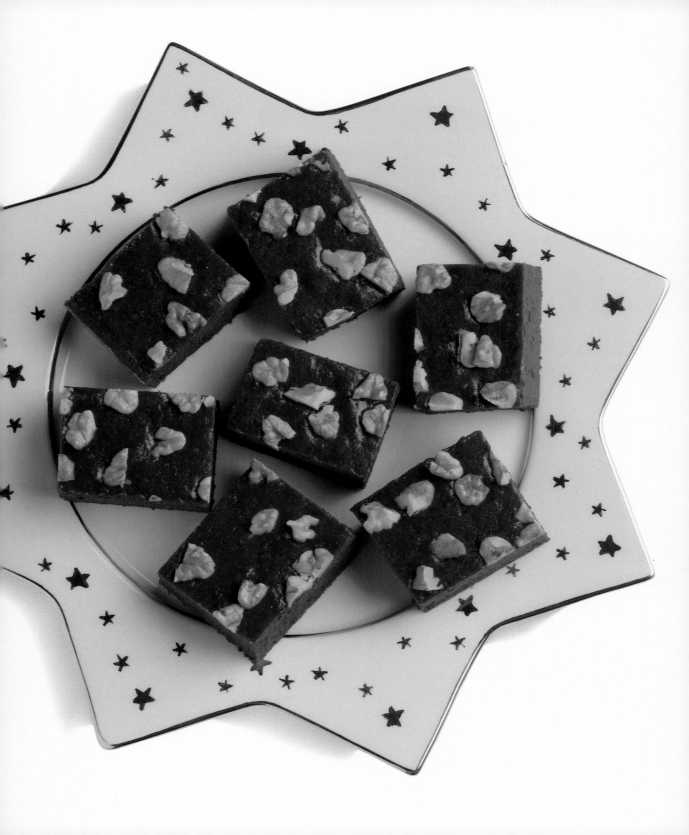

Serve these crisp, lowfat Italian cookies—their name means "twice-baked"—
with coffee or the Tuscan dessert wine known as *vin santo*. Store in a tightly covered
container for up to a month; their taste improves with a day or two of storage.

Anise Biscotti

Makes 4 dozen cookies

2 cups (10 oz/315 g) all-purpose
(plain) flour
2 teaspoons baking powder
⅛ teaspoon sea salt
¼ cup (1 oz/30 g) slivered
almonds, toasted

2 tablespoons unsalted butter, at
room temperature
¾ cup (6 oz/185 g) sugar
1 teaspoon almond extract (essence)
1 teaspoon fresh lemon juice
1 tablespoon aniseeds
3 egg whites, lightly beaten

1. Preheat an oven to 325°F (165°C). Coat a large baking sheet
with nonstick cooking spray.
2. In a medium bowl, stir together the flour, baking powder
and salt. Add the toasted almonds and stir to mix well.
3. In a large bowl, using an electric mixer set on medium speed,
beat together the butter and sugar until light and creamy,
2–3 minutes. Add the almond extract, lemon juice and aniseeds
and beat until combined. Using a rubber spatula, stir in the egg
whites. Then, with the mixer set on low speed, beat in the flour
mixture until the ingredients come together to form a ball,
about 1 minute.
4. Turn out the dough onto a lightly floured work surface and
divide in half. Using your palms, shape each half into a log
about 9 inches (23 cm) long and 2 inches (5 cm) wide. Transfer
each log to the prepared baking sheet. Press down on the tops
of the logs to flatten slightly, to give the biscotti their distinctive
look once they are cut and baked.
5. Bake until the dough is firm and a toothpick inserted into
the center comes out clean, about 20 minutes. Remove from
the oven to cool for a few minutes.

*Nutritional Analysis
Per Cookie:*

Calories 47
(Kilojoules 196)
Protein 1 g
Carbohydrates 8 g
Total Fat 1 g
Saturated Fat 0 g
Cholesterol 1 mg
Sodium 28 mg
Dietary Fiber 0 g

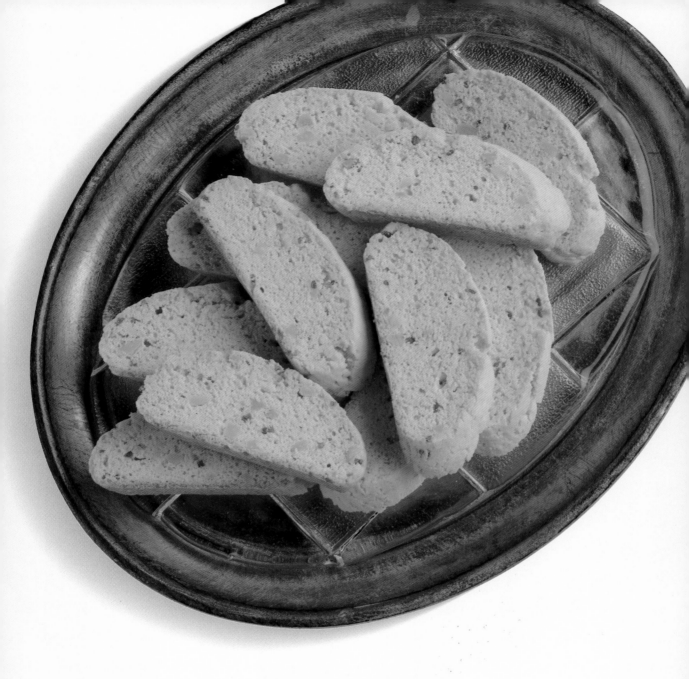

6. Reduce the oven temperature to 250°F (120°C). While the logs are still warm, using a serrated knife, cut them diagonally into slices ½ inch (12 mm) thick. Lay the slices, cut-side down, on 2 baking sheets and return them to the oven. Bake until the slices are crisp and golden, 8–15 minutes. Transfer to a rack to cool completely before serving or storing.

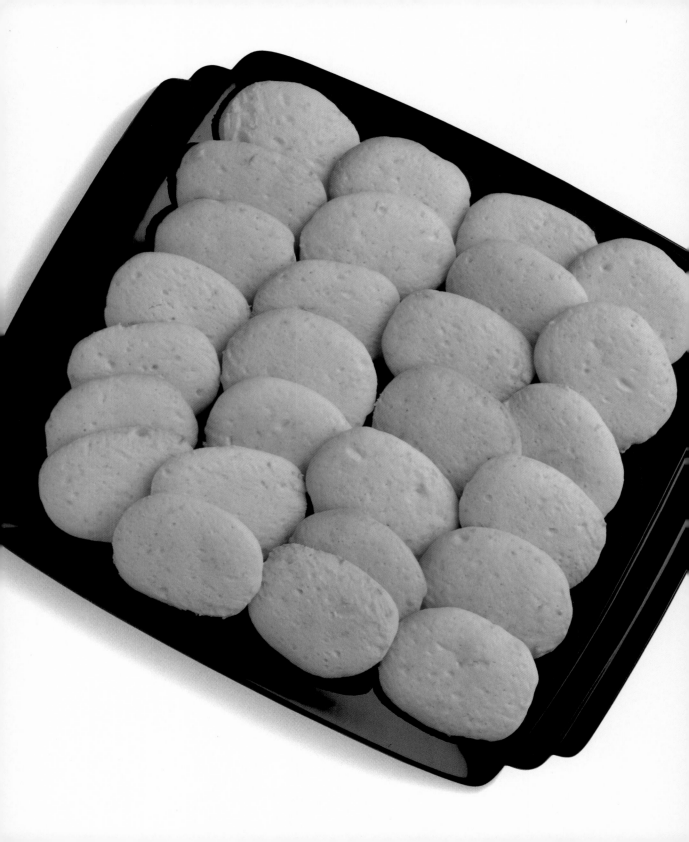

Icebox cookie doughs require chilling to make them firm enough to slice for baking. The dough keeps in the refrigerator for up to 1 week and in the freezer up to 1 month. Whenever you want cookies, just slice off as many as you need from the log.

Lemon Icebox Cookies

Makes 30 cookies

1¾ cups (9 oz/280 g) all-purpose (plain) flour
1 teaspoon baking powder
6 tablespoons (3 fl oz/90 ml) vegetable oil or melted unsalted butter

⅓ cup (3 oz/90 g) Vanilla Sugar *(recipe on page 125)* or granulated sugar
grated zest of 2 lemons
2 tablespoons fresh lemon juice
2 eggs
⅟₁₆ teaspoon salt

1. In a bowl, stir together the flour and baking powder. Set aside.
2. In a food processor fitted with the metal blade, combine the vegetable oil or butter and the Vanilla Sugar or granulated sugar. Process until creamy, about 20 seconds. Add the lemon zest, lemon juice, eggs and salt and process until well blended. Add the flour mixture and pulse a few times just to incorporate. Alternatively, in a bowl, using an electric mixer set on medium speed, beat together the oil or butter and the Vanilla Sugar until creamy, 2–3 minutes. Beat in the lemon zest, lemon juice, eggs and salt and beat until combined. Reduce the speed to low and beat in the flour mixture until incorporated.
3. Spoon the dough onto a sheet of waxed paper. Using your hands, shape the dough into a log 2 inches (5 cm) in diameter. Cover and refrigerate for a minimum of 2 hours prior to baking.
4. Preheat an oven to 350°F (180°C).
5. Unwrap the dough; place on a work surface. Using a sharp knife, cut the dough into slices ¼ inch (6 mm) thick. Place them on an ungreased baking sheet. Bake just until the cookies begin to color and are firm in the center, about 10 minutes. Transfer to a rack to cool completely before serving or storing.
6. Store in a tightly covered container for up to 2 weeks.

Nutritional Analysis Per Cookie:

**Calories 70
(Kilojoules 295)
Protein 1 g
Carbohydrates 9 g
Total Fat 3 g
Saturated Fat 0 g
Cholesterol 14 mg
Sodium 25 mg
Dietary Fiber 0 g**

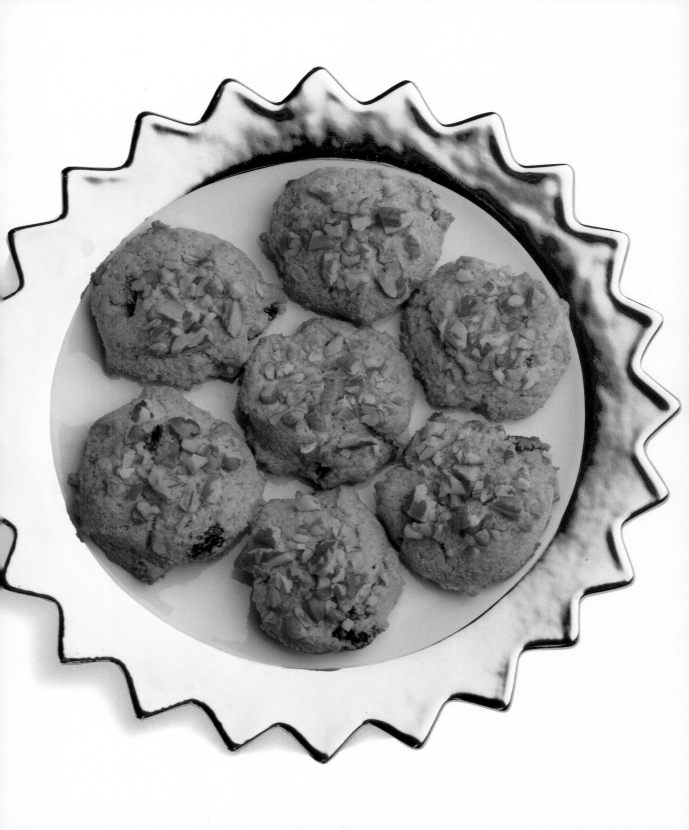

A specialty of Cape Cod, Massachusetts, hermits were originally developed to be taken on long sea voyages, because they stay fresh and chewy a long time. This version reduces the fat traditionally used, but the cookies' flavor and texture remain unchanged.

Whole-Wheat Hermit Cookies

Makes 2 dozen cookies

½ cup (3½ oz/105 g) firmly packed brown sugar

½ cup (4 oz/125 g) unsalted butter, chilled and sliced

1 egg

½ cup (4 fl oz/125 ml) nonfat sour cream

2 cups (10 oz/315 g) whole-wheat (wholemeal) flour

¼ teaspoon baking powder

1 teaspoon ground cinnamon

¼ teaspoon baking soda (bicarbonate of soda)

½ cup (3 oz/90 g) raisins

½ cup (2 oz/60 g) finely chopped walnuts or pecans

1. Preheat an oven to 350°F (180°C). Coat 2 baking sheets with nonstick cooking spray.

2. In a large bowl, using an electric mixer set on medium speed, beat together the brown sugar and butter until light and creamy, 2–3 minutes. Add the egg and sour cream and beat until well combined.

3. In a medium bowl, stir together the flour, baking powder, cinnamon, baking soda and raisins. Stir the flour mixture into the sugar mixture until thoroughly incorporated.

4. Drop the dough by the teaspoonful onto the prepared baking sheets, spacing the cookies about 3 inches (7.5 cm) apart. Sprinkle the walnuts or pecans over the top. Bake until brown and firm, 12–15 minutes. Transfer to a rack to cool completely before serving or storing.

5. Store in a tightly covered container for several weeks.

Nutritional Analysis Per Cookie:

Calories 123
(Kilojoules 515)
Protein 3 g
Carbohydrates 16 g
Total Fat 6 g
Saturated Fat 3 g
Cholesterol 19 mg
Sodium 27 mg
Dietary Fiber 2 g

Molasses and ginger combine to give these crisp cookies their distinctive fragrance. Fresh ginger, if you can find it, provides the most aroma and flavor, but ground ginger also produces excellent results.

Gingersnaps

Makes 18 cookies

2 tablespoons unsalted butter, at room temperature

¼ cup (2 oz/60 g) firmly packed brown sugar

1 egg, lightly beaten

½ cup (6 oz/185 g) light molasses, dark corn syrup or honey

2 tablespoons vegetable oil

1 piece fresh ginger, 1 inch (2.5 cm) long, peeled and grated, or 1 teaspoon ground ginger

1½ cups (7½ oz/235 g) all-purpose (plain) flour

1 teaspoon ground cinnamon

¼ teaspoon ground cloves

1 teaspoon baking soda (bicarbonate of soda)

¼ cup (2 fl oz/60 ml) lowfat buttermilk

6 tablespoons (3 fl oz/90 ml) Ricotta Icing *(recipe on page 124)*, optional

1. Preheat an oven to 375°F (190°C). Coat a large baking sheet with nonstick cooking spray.

2. In a food processor fitted with the metal blade, combine the butter and brown sugar. Process until light and creamy, about 20 seconds. Add the egg, molasses or other liquid sweetener, oil and ginger and process until blended, about 30 seconds. Alternatively, in a medium bowl, using an electric mixer set on medium speed, beat together the butter and sugar until light and creamy, 2–3 minutes. Add the egg, molasses or other liquid sweetener, oil and ginger and beat until combined, 2–3 minutes.

3. In a large bowl, stir together the flour, cinnamon, cloves and baking soda. Spoon the creamed mixture into the flour mixture, and stir until well combined. Stir in the buttermilk.

4. Drop the dough by the teaspoonful onto the prepared baking sheet, spacing about 3 inches (7.5 cm) apart. Dampen your fingers with warm water and shape each ball into a

Nutritional Analysis Per Cookie:

Calories 111

(Kilojoules 467)

Protein 2 g

Carbohydrates 19 g

Total Fat 3 g

Saturated Fat 1 g

Cholesterol 15 mg

Sodium 82 mg

Dietary Fiber 0 g

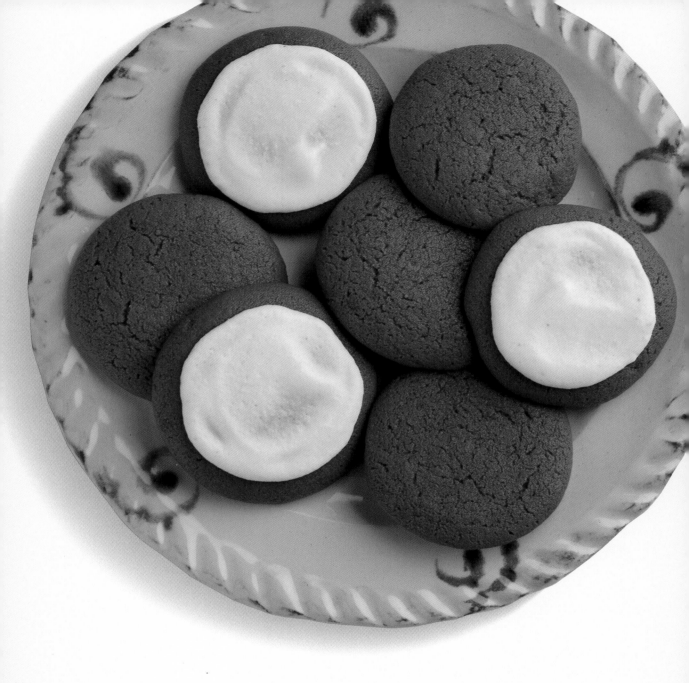

flattened disk about ¼ inch (6 mm) thick. Bake until the cookies are set and the tops are cracked, about 12 minutes. Transfer to a rack to cool completely before serving or storing.

5. Ice the cookies with the Ricotta Icing, if using. Store in a tightly covered container for 1 week.

This rich-tasting dessert makes excellent use of good bread that's a day or two old. The molasses, vanilla and bourbon produce a satisfying flavor for the light custard mixture in which the bread soaks. A little more bourbon flavors the topping.

BOURBON BREAD PUDDING

Serves 10

½ lb (250 g) day-old French bread, crusts removed and bread cut into slices ½ inch (12 mm) thick

3 cups (24 fl oz/750 ml) lowfat buttermilk

2 eggs

1 cup (8 oz/250 g) sugar

¼ cup (3 oz/90 g) molasses

1 teaspoon vanilla extract (essence)

4 tablespoons (2 fl oz/60 ml) bourbon (whisky)

½ cup (3 oz/90 g) raisins

¼ teaspoon ground cinnamon

¾ cup (6 fl oz/180 ml) Lowfat Crème Anglaise *(recipe on page 127)* or lowfat plain yogurt

1. Preheat an oven to 350°F (180°C). Coat a 9-inch (23-cm) loaf pan with nonstick cooking spray.

2. Place the bread slices in a shallow bowl and pour the buttermilk over them. Let stand until the bread soaks up the buttermilk and is soft, 15 minutes.

3. In another bowl, stir together the eggs, sugar, molasses, vanilla extract and half of the bourbon.

4. Place half of the softened bread slices in the loaf pan. Scatter the raisins over the bread. Top with the remaining bread slices in a single layer. Pour the egg mixture evenly over the top and sprinkle with the cinnamon. Bake until golden brown, 30–40 minutes.

5. Stir the remaining bourbon into the Lowfat Crème Anglaise or yogurt.

6. To serve, scoop the pudding into individual bowls, top each serving with an equal amount of the Crème Anglaise mixture.

Nutritional Analysis Per Serving:

CALORIES 265
(KILOJOULES 1,112)
PROTEIN 6 G
CARBOHYDRATES 53 G
TOTAL FAT 3 G
SATURATED FAT 1 G
CHOLESTEROL 53 MG
SODIUM 227 MG
DIETARY FIBER 1 G

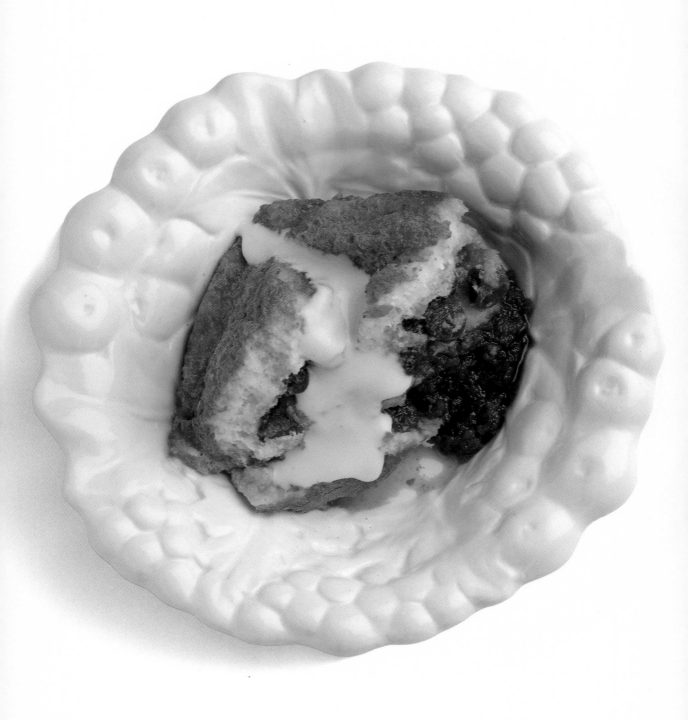

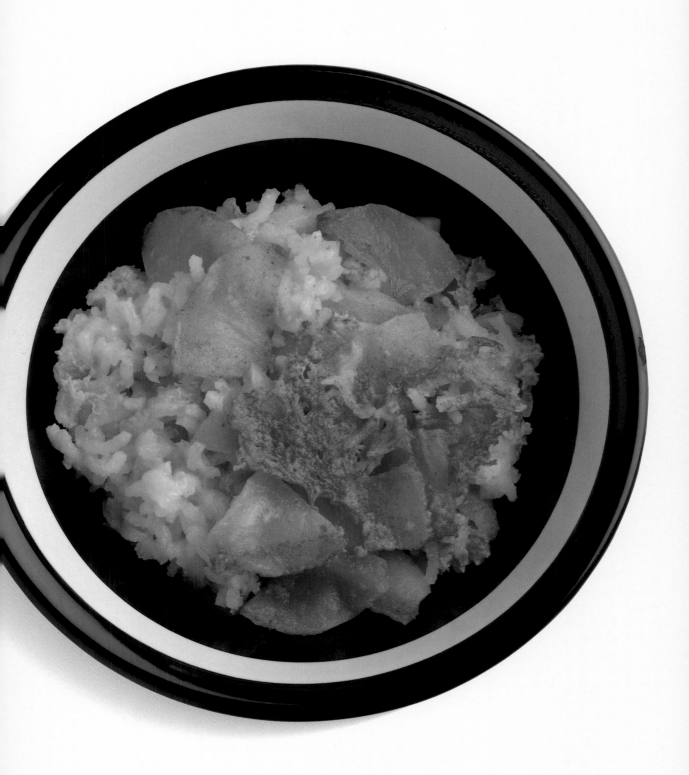

Basmati rice from India or the United States or jasmine rice from Thailand adds a wonderful fragrance to this recipe, but any long-grained variety works well. You can substitute slices of peach, mango or fig for the apple. The recipe doubles beautifully.

Fragrant Rice Pudding

Serves 6

2 tablespoons unsalted butter

5 tablespoons (3 oz/90 g) sugar

2 large cooking apples such as York, Gala or Jonathan, 1 lb (500 g) total weight, quartered, cored, peeled and thinly sliced

1 teaspoon ground cinnamon

½ cup (3½ oz/105 g) basmati or jasmine rice

2 cups (16 fl oz/500 ml) lowfat (1%) milk

1. Preheat an oven to 350°F (180°C).

2. In a 12-inch (30-cm) cast-iron frying pan or flameproof 2-qt (2-l) baking dish over medium heat, combine the butter and 2 tablespoons of the sugar. When the mixture is hot and bubbling, add the apples and sauté, stirring, until soft and fragrant, about 5 minutes. Add half of the cinnamon to the fruit as it cooks.

3. Meanwhile, in a bowl, combine the rice, milk, the remaining 3 tablespoons of sugar and the remaining cinnamon. Stir to mix well.

4. When the apples are soft, pour the rice mixture evenly over the top. Cover with a lid or aluminum foil and bake until the milk has thickened and the rice is tender and small holes have formed in the top, 1½–2 hours. Do not stir during the last half of cooking.

5. To serve, scoop into individual bowls.

Nutritional Analysis Per Serving:

CALORIES 216
(KILOJOULES 907)
PROTEIN 5 G
CARBOHYDRATES 41 G
TOTAL FAT 5 G
SATURATED FAT 3 G
CHOLESTEROL 14 MG
SODIUM 49 MG
DIETARY FIBER 1 G

Made in the classic fashion with egg whites only, virtually fat-free baked meringues add a touch of healthy elegance to dessert. Fill these with whatever fresh berries are in season, such as strawberries, raspberries, blackberries or blueberries.

Meringues & Berries with Lemon Sauce

Serves 6

4 egg whites, at room temperature

1 cup (7 oz/220 g) superfine (caster) sugar

1 teaspoon vanilla extract (essence)

1 teaspoon distilled white vinegar

6 tablespoons (3 fl oz/90 ml) Lemon Sauce *(recipe on page 74)*

2 cups (8 oz/250 g) berries

mint leaves

Nutritional Analysis Per Serving:

CALORIES 191
(KILOJOULES 804)
PROTEIN 3 G
CARBOHYDRATES 42 G
TOTAL FAT 2 G
SATURATED FAT 1 G
CHOLESTEROL 5 MG
SODIUM 43 MG
DIETARY FIBER 1 G

1. Preheat the oven to 250°F (120°C). Line a baking sheet with parchment paper.

2. In a clean bowl, using an electric mixer set on high speed, beat the egg whites until stiff peaks form. Slowly add the sugar, beating on high continuously. Add the vanilla and vinegar. Beat until extremely stiff, 5–7 minutes.

3. Using a large spoon, form 6 mounds of egg white mixture on the baking sheet. With the back of the spoon, form an indentation in the center of each mound.

4. Bake until the meringues are pinkish beige, about 1 hour. To test that the meringues are ready, gently touch the bottom of each indentation with your fingertip. If it is sticky, bake a few minutes longer.

5. Using a metal spatula, lift the meringues off the baking sheet the moment they are removed from the oven and transfer to a piece of waxed paper or directly onto individual plates. (If they sit even a few seconds, they will crack and break.)

6. To serve, fill each meringue with 1 tablespoon of the Lemon Sauce and top each with an equal amount of berries. Garnish with the mint leaves.

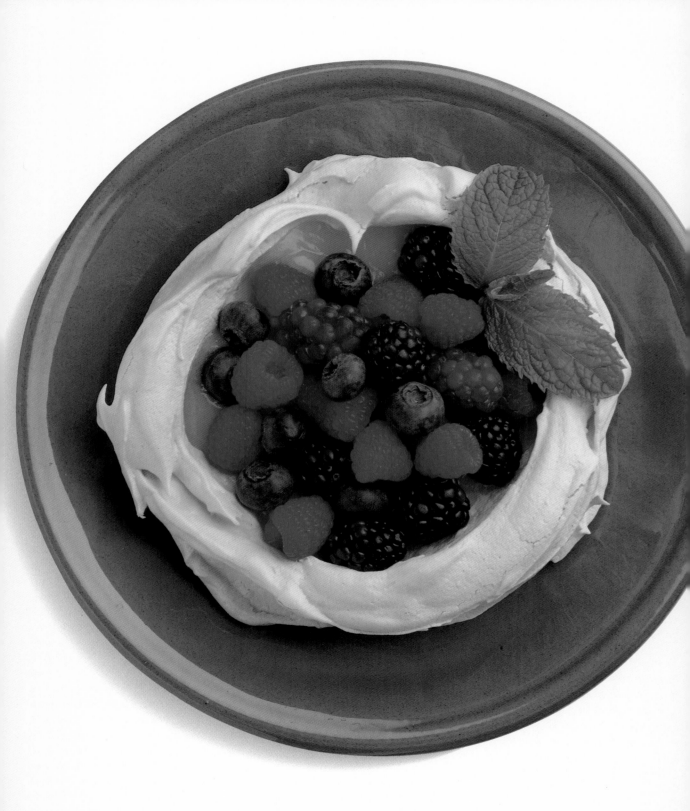

The classic Italian pastry shells known as cannoli are fried before filling with sweetened ricotta cheese and candied fruit. These crisp crêpes have a similar texture, resulting from the inclusion of crunchy wheat germ and a short stint in the oven.

Chocolate Cannoli with Sweetened Yogurt

Serves 12

¼ cup (1½ oz/45 g) all-purpose
 (plain) flour
1 tablespoon unsweetened cocoa
2 tablespoons granulated sugar
2 tablespoons toasted wheat germ
⅓ cup (3 fl oz/80 ml) nonfat milk
2 egg whites
1 teaspoon almond extract (essence)
1–2 tablespoons water
1 tablespoon confectioners' (icing)
 sugar for dusting

Sweetened Yogurt
½ cup (3 oz/90 g) candied fruit,
 finely chopped, optional
2 tablespoons Marsala wine or
 dry sherry, if using candied fruit
1½ cups (12 oz/375 g) Yogurt Cheese
 (recipe on page 124) or lowfat
 ricotta cheese
1 tablespoon confectioners' (icing)
 sugar, sifted after measuring

*Nutritional Analysis
Per Serving:*

Calories 81
(Kilojoules 340)
Protein 4 g
Carbohydrates 13 g
Total Fat 1 g
Saturated Fat 0 g
Cholesterol 1 mg
Sodium 31 mg
Dietary Fiber 0 g

1. Prepare the Sweetened Yogurt (see opposite page).
2. In a bowl, sift together the flour and cocoa. Stir in the granulated sugar and wheat germ. In another bowl, using a whisk, stir together the milk, egg whites and almond extract. Whisk the milk mixture into the flour mixture. Let stand for 20 minutes. The batter will thicken upon standing. Add the water and stir again to mix well.
3. Preheat an oven to 500°F (260°C).
4. Place an 8-inch (20-cm) nonstick frying pan over medium-high heat. When hot, coat with nonstick cooking spray and reduce the heat to medium–low. Spoon in 2 tablespoons of batter and swirl the pan to spread the batter to form a round 3 inches (7.5 cm) in diameter. If the batter won't spread to the desired size, stir another tablespoon water into the bowl of batter. Cook each crêpe until bubbles form on the top and the edges are firm, about 20 seconds. If the crêpe begins to scorch, reduce the heat. Flip over the crêpe and cook until lightly browned, 10–15 seconds longer.

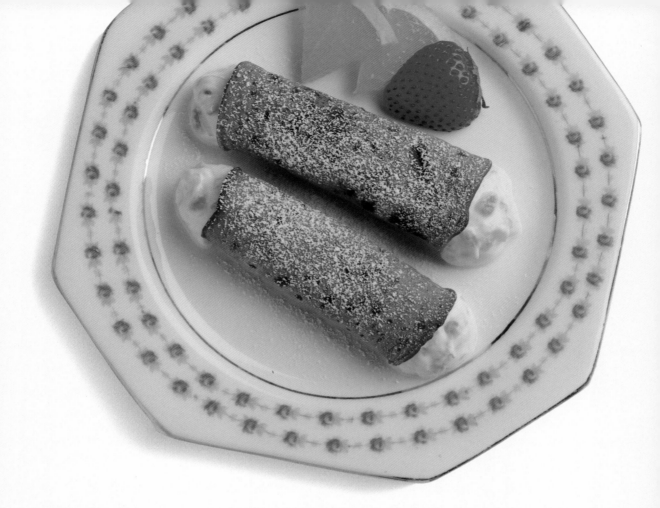

5. Transfer the crêpe to an ungreased baking sheet and roll up into a cylinder 1 inch (2.5 cm) in diameter. Lay the crêpe, seam-side down, on the baking sheet and continue to make the remaining crêpes. As each crêpe is cooked, roll it up and place it on the baking sheet.

6. When all the crêpes are made, place them in the oven just until the edges are crisp and the middle of each crêpe turns slightly brittle, about 5 minutes. If you leave them any longer, they will toughen. Remove from the oven to cool.

7. To serve, spoon the Sweetened Yogurt into a pastry bag fitted with a large round tip. Pipe into the cooled shells. Lay the filled shells side by side on a large serving platter and dust with the confectioners' sugar.

SWEETENED YOGURT

1. In a shallow bowl, combine the candied fruit and Marsala or sherry, if using, and let stand until the liquid is absorbed, about 15 minutes. The sticky pieces of fruit should now separate easily and be gleaming. If any liquid remains, drain the fruit on a paper towel. Stir in the Yogurt Cheese or ricotta and confectioners' sugar.

2. Refrigerate the mixture until ready to use. The filling will keep for several hours.

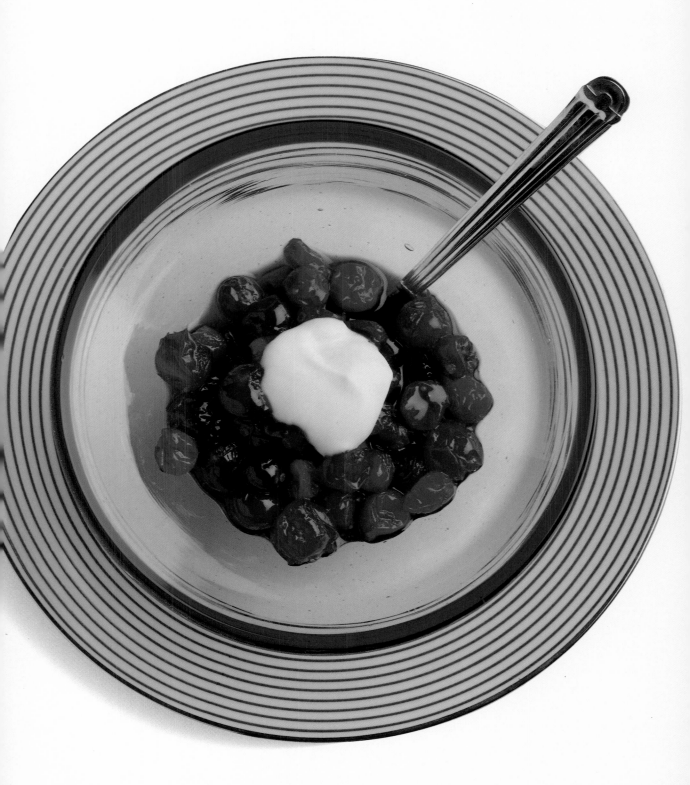

A splash of ruby port adds an almost chocolatey flavor to this dessert, which is excellent in late autumn when fresh cranberries are available. In other seasons, use widely available frozen whole cranberries.

Baked Cranberries

Serves 10

3 cups (12 oz/375 g) fresh or frozen cranberries
1 cup (7 oz/220 g) firmly packed brown sugar
2 tablespoons fresh orange juice

grated zest of 1 orange
¼ cup (2 fl oz/60 ml) port wine or balsamic vinegar
¾ cup (6 fl oz/180 ml) nonfat sour cream

1. Preheat an oven to 300°F (150°C).
2. In a 1–qt (1–l) baking dish, combine the cranberries, brown sugar and orange juice and zest. Stir to mix well. Cover and bake until the cranberries are dark and the juice is bubbling, about 1 hour.
3. Stir in the port or vinegar, cover and let stand at room temperature to cool.
4. To serve, spoon into individual bowls. Top each serving with an equal amount of sour cream.

Nutritional Analysis Per Serving:

Calories 115
(Kilojoules 484)
Protein 1 g
Carbohydrates 26 g
Total Fat 0 g
Saturated Fat 0 g
Cholesterol 0 mg
Sodium 21 mg
Dietary Fiber 0 g

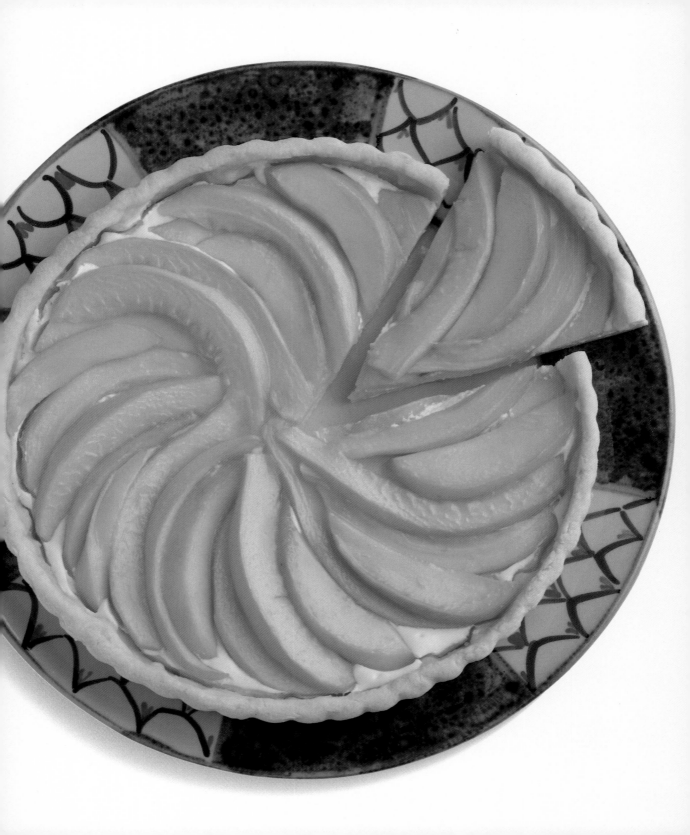

Slices of two widely available tropical fruits yield an eye-catching,
easily made tart for spring or summer. The Neufchâtel cream cheese used
in the filling adds rich flavor to the tart with little additional fat.

Mango & Papaya Tart

Serves 8

Lowfat Pastry *(recipe on page 126)*
  or other 9-inch (23-cm)
  pie crust
½ cup (4 oz/125 g) Yogurt Cheese
  (recipe on page 124)
3 oz (90 g) Neufchâtel cheese,
  at room temperature

1 tablespoon Vanilla Sugar *(recipe on page 125)* or granulated sugar
1 ripe mango, ¾ lb (375 g), halved, pitted, peeled and sliced
1 ripe papaya, 1 lb (500 g), halved, seeded, peeled and sliced
2 tablespoons fresh lime juice

1. Preheat an oven to 375°F (190°C). Roll out the Lowfat
Pastry and line a 9-inch (23-cm) tart pan with a removable
bottom, then partially bake as directed. Let cool completely.
2. In a food processor fitted with the metal blade, combine
the Yogurt Cheese, Neufchâtel cheese and Vanilla Sugar or
granulated sugar and process until well blended, 10–20 seconds.
Alternatively, using a wooden spoon or a whisk, beat together
all the ingredients in a bowl.
3. Spread the cheese mixture into the cooled pie shell. Arrange
the mango and papaya slices in concentric circles on top. Sprinkle
the lime juice over the fruit. Bake until the fruit is soft and juicy,
15–20 minutes. Transfer to a rack to cool completely, about
20 minutes.
4. To serve, cut into wedges and place on individual plates.

Nutritional Analysis Per Serving:

**Calories 225
(Kilojoules 945)
Protein 6 g
Carbohydrates 35 g
Total Fat 7 g
Saturated Fat 3 g
Cholesterol 12 mg
Sodium 95 mg
Dietary Fiber 1 g**

Made with less fat than conventional doughs, the biscuits for this cobbler can also be used for strawberry shortcake or, if the sugar is omitted, for dinner biscuits. Fat is further reduced by omitting the butter typically layered between fruit and dough.

Blueberry & Peach Cobbler

Serves 8

8 large very ripe peaches, 4 lb (2 kg) total weight, halved, pitted, peeled and sliced
1 cup (4 oz/125 g) blueberries
¼ cup (2 oz/60 g) sugar
½ teaspoon ground cinnamon

Biscuit Dough

1 cup (5 oz/155 g) all-purpose (plain) flour
1/16 teaspoon salt
2 tablespoons sugar
1 teaspoon baking powder
3 tablespoons unsalted butter or vegetable shortening
5 tablespoons (3 fl oz/80 ml) lowfat milk

Nutritional Analysis Per Serving:

Calories 231
(Kilojoules 968)
Protein 3 g
Carbohydrates 46 g
Total Fat 5 g
Saturated Fat 3 g
Cholesterol 12 mg
Sodium 84 mg
Dietary Fiber 4 g

1. Prepare the Biscuit Dough (see below).
2. Preheat an oven to 425°F (220°C). Coat an 8-inch (20-cm) square baking pan with nonstick cooking spray.
3. Combine the peaches and berries in the bottom of the prepared pan. Sprinkle on the sugar and cinnamon.
4. Lay the Biscuit Dough squares in a single layer on top of the fruit in the pan.
5. Bake until the biscuit topping is golden brown and puffy and the fruit juices are bubbling up around the edges, about 35 minutes.
6. To serve, using a large spoon, scoop squares of dough with fruit and juices into individual bowls.

Biscuit Dough

1. In a food processor fitted with the metal blade, combine the flour, salt, sugar and baking powder and pulse to combine. Add the butter or shortening and pulse just until the mixture resembles small peas, about 5 seconds. With the motor running, add the milk in a thin, steady stream, and process only until the dough begins to form a ball. Alternatively, to make the dough by hand, stir together the dry ingredients in a bowl. Add the butter or shortening and, using your fingers or a pastry blender, work the ingredients together until the mixture resembles small peas. Using a fork, stir in the milk and continue to stir and toss until the mixture starts to form a ball.
2. Transfer the dough to a floured work surface and knead 5 times. Roll out the dough to ½–¾ inch (12 mm–2 cm) thick. Cut the dough into 8 equal squares.

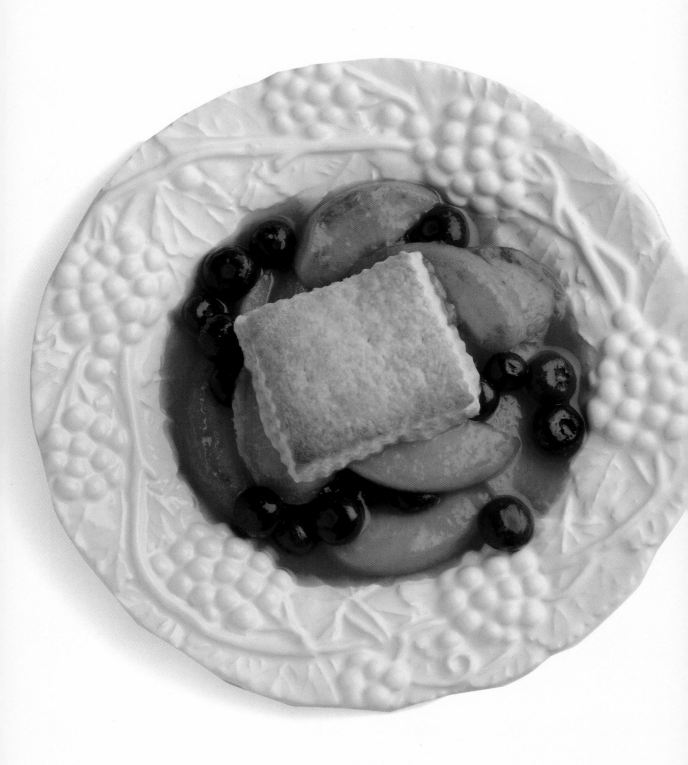

*J*ust a little butter and nuts in the topping gives this crisp plenty
of taste and texture. Choose pears that are neither too juicy nor too soft, such as
Bartlett (Williams'). The self-formed pastry provides an interesting presentation.

*P*EAR CRISP

Serves 8

Lowfat Pastry *(recipe on page 126)* or
    other 9-inch (23-cm) pie crust
2 tablespoons apricot fruit spread
3 firm, ripe pears, ¾ lb (375 g)
    total weight, quartered, cored,
    peeled and thinly sliced

½ cup (1½ oz/45 g) graham cracker
    crumbs (2 full-size crackers)
2 walnuts, shelled
3 tablespoons firmly packed brown sugar
½ teaspoon ground cinnamon
1 tablespoon unsalted butter
1 teaspoon crystallized ginger, chopped

1. Preheat an oven to 425°F (220°C).

2. On a piece of floured aluminum foil on a work surface, roll
out the Lowfat Pastry into a 10-inch (25-cm) round. Turn up
the edges of the dough to form a rim about 1½ inches (4 cm)
high. Flute the edge. Bring up the foil to hold up the sides of the
dough. Slide the pastry and foil onto an ungreased baking sheet.

3. In a small saucepan over medium heat, melt the fruit spread
until it liquefies, about 1 minute. Brush the bottom of the pastry
with the liquid.

4. Arrange the pear slices, overlapping them, in concentric circles
over the bottom of the pastry. Trim any leftover slices as needed
to fill the center.

5. In a food processor fitted with the metal blade, combine the
graham crackers and walnuts and process to chop finely, 5–10
seconds. Add the brown sugar and cinnamon and pulse a few
times. Add the butter and pulse just to incorporate it. Sprinkle
the cracker mixture evenly over the pears. Dot with the
crystallized ginger.

6. Bake for 10 minutes. Reduce the heat to 350°F (180°C)
and bake until the pears are soft when pierced and the pastry is

*Nutritional Analysis
Per Serving:*

**CALORIES 235
(KILOJOULES 985)
PROTEIN 3 G
CARBOHYDRATES 40 G
TOTAL FAT 7 G
SATURATED FAT 2 G
CHOLESTEROL 7 MG
SODIUM 78 MG
DIETARY FIBER 1 G**

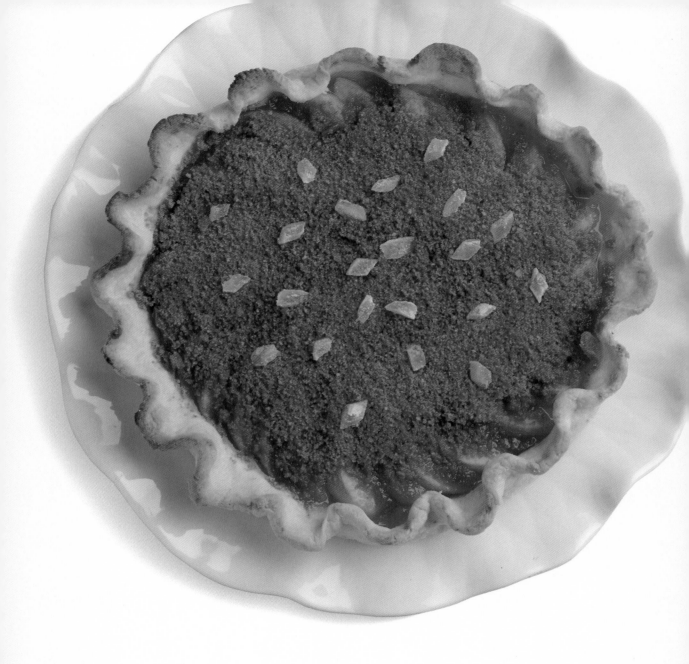

golden, about 15 minutes longer. If the pastry begins to brown
too much before the pears are tender, cover with additional
aluminum foil. Leaving on the baking sheet, transfer to a rack
to cool completely, about 20 minutes.

7. To serve, carefully slide the crisp onto a serving plate and
cut into wedges.

A classic pie filling of pumpkin, rich in potassium and vitamin A, becomes extra healthy in this lowfat variation made with buttermilk, which has a tanginess that nicely complements the natural sweetness of the squash.

Pumpkin Pie

Serves 8

Lowfat Pastry *(recipe on page 126)*
  or other 9-inch (23-cm) pie crust
1 can (14½ oz/455 g) pumpkin
  purée
1½ cups (12 fl oz/375 ml) lowfat
  buttermilk
½ cup (4 oz/125 g) granulated
  sugar
½ cup (3½ oz/105 g) firmly
  packed brown sugar
½ teaspoon ground cinnamon
½ teaspoon ground allspice
¹⁄₁₆ teaspoon ground cloves

1. Preheat an oven to 425°F (220°C). Roll out the Lowfat Pastry and line a 9-inch (23-cm) pie pan. Place the pie pan on a baking sheet and set aside.
2. In a bowl, using a wooden spoon, stir together the pumpkin and buttermilk until well combined. Stir in the granulated and brown sugars, cinnamon, allspice and cloves.
3. Pour the filling into the pie shell. Bake for 10 minutes. Reduce the oven temperature to 350°F (180°C) and bake until the top is set, 35 minutes longer. Transfer to a rack to cool completely, about 30 minutes.
4. To serve, cut into wedges and place on plates.

Nutritional Analysis Per Serving:

Calories 274
(Kilojoules 1,150)
Protein 5 g
Carbohydrates 54 g
Total Fat 5 g
Saturated Fat 2 g
Cholesterol 5 mg
Sodium 97 mg
Dietary Fiber 1 g

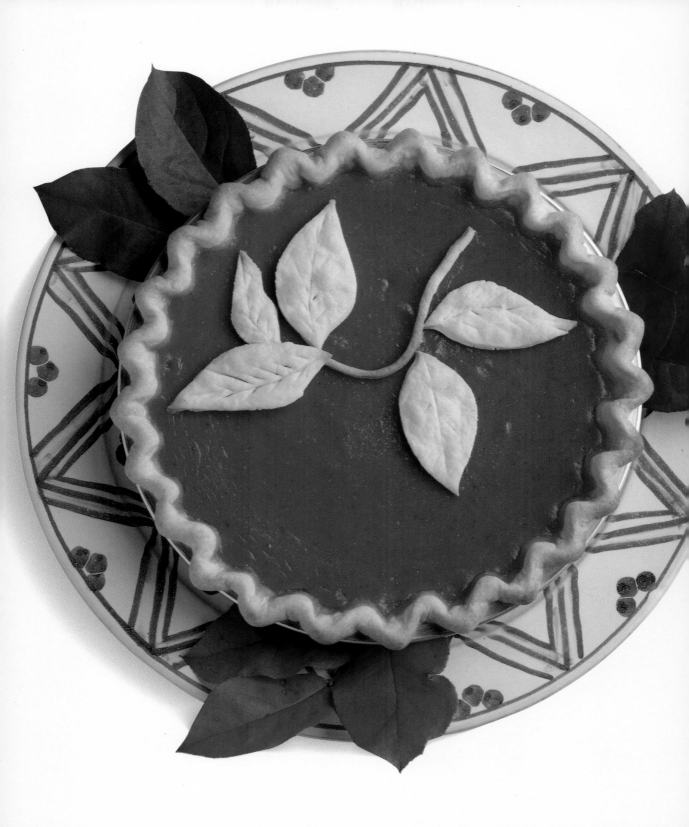

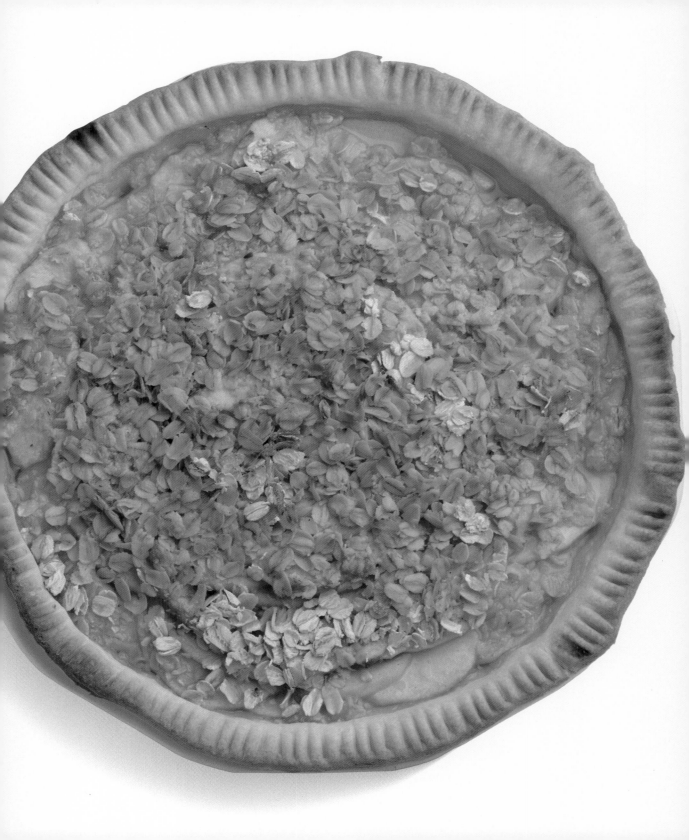

A crumb topping cuts the amount of pastry in half, and therefore raises the proportion of healthy apples per serving. Choose an apple variety that holds its shape well during cooking and has a spicy flavor, such as Granny Smith, Gala, Jonagold, Empire or York.

CRUMB-TOPPED APPLE PIE

Serves 8

Lowfat Pastry *(recipe on page 126)*
  or other 9-inch (23-cm) pie crust
2 lb (1 kg) apples, quartered, cored,
  peeled and thinly sliced
2 tablespoons fresh lemon juice
2 tablespoons all-purpose
  (plain) flour

¾ cup (6 oz/185 g) sugar
1/16 teaspoon salt
½ teaspoon ground cinnamon
¾ cup (2 oz/60 g) lowfat muesli
  or rolled oats
2 tablespoons unsalted butter,
  chilled and cut into 8 pieces

1. Preheat an oven to 400°F (200°C). Roll out the Lowfat Pastry and line a 9-inch (23-cm) pie pan. Place the pie pan on a baking sheet and set aside.
2. Sprinkle the apples with the lemon juice and set aside.
3. In a large bowl, using a whisk, stir together the flour, sugar, salt and cinnamon.
4. Add the apples to the flour mixture and toss to mix well. Spread into the pie shell. Top with the muesli or rolled oats and dot with the butter.
5. Bake until the crumbs are golden brown, 45–50 minutes. Transfer to a rack to cool completely, about 20 minutes.
6. To serve, cut into wedges and place on individual plates.

Nutritional Analysis Per Serving:

**CALORIES 334
(KILOJOULES 1,403)
PROTEIN 4 G
CARBOHYDRATES 64 G
TOTAL FAT 8 G
SATURATED FAT 3 G
CHOLESTEROL 11 MG
SODIUM 72 MG
DIETARY FIBER 2 G**

The tang of the lowfat buttermilk in the batter highlights the spicy fragrance of the fresh ginger. The light sauce made with lemon juice and zest—and a little butter—transforms this homey cake into a special dessert.

Gingerbread with Lemon Sauce

Serves 12

1½ cups (7½ oz/235 g) all-purpose (plain) flour
1½ teaspoons baking powder
½ teaspoon salt
¼ cup (2 oz/60 g) unsalted butter, at room temperature
¼ cup (2 fl oz/60 ml) vegetable oil
½ cup (3 ½ oz/105 g) firmly packed brown sugar
½ cup (6 oz/185 g) honey
1 egg
½ cup (4 fl oz/125 ml) lowfat buttermilk
1 piece fresh ginger, 1 inch (2.5 cm) long, peeled and grated

Nutritional Analysis Per Serving:

CALORIES 301
(KILOJOULES 1,264)
PROTEIN 3 G
CARBOHYDRATES 45 G
TOTAL FAT 13 G
SATURATED FAT 6 G
CHOLESTEROL 39 MG
SODIUM 184 MG
DIETARY FIBER 0 G

LEMON SAUCE

½ cup (4 oz/125 g) sugar
2 tablespoons cornstarch (cornflour)
1/16 teaspoon salt
2 cups (16 fl oz/500 ml) water
¼ cup (2 oz/60 g) unsalted butter
1 tablespoon grated lemon zest
3 tablespoons fresh lemon juice

1. Preheat an oven to 350°F (180°C). Coat an 8-inch (20-cm) square pan with nonstick cooking spray.
2. In a bowl, stir together the flour, baking powder and salt.
3. In a food processor fitted with the metal blade, combine the butter, vegetable oil and brown sugar. Process until creamy, 10–20 seconds. Add the honey and egg and process until smooth, 1 minute. Process in the flour mixture, buttermilk and ginger briefly. Alternatively, in a large bowl, using an electric mixer set on medium speed, beat together the butter, oil and brown sugar until creamy, 2–3 minutes. Add the honey and egg and beat until smooth. Stir in the flour mixture, buttermilk and ginger.
4. Pour the batter into the prepared pan. Bake until golden brown and the edges start to separate from the pan, 35–40 minutes. The cake will have a soft texture, but a toothpick inserted in the center should come out clean.
5. Prepare the Lemon Sauce (see opposite page).

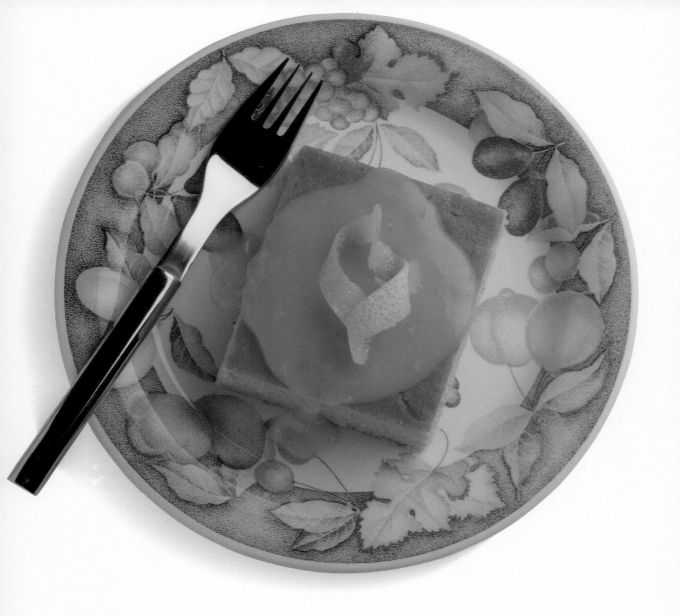

6. To serve, cut the warm cake into squares and place on individual plates. Top each serving with 2 tablespoons of Lemon Sauce.

LEMON SAUCE

1. In a saucepan, stir together the sugar, cornstarch and salt. Stir in the water and place over medium heat. Cook, stirring constantly, until the mixture boils and thickens, about 4 minutes.

2. Remove from the heat and stir in the butter and the lemon zest and juice. This recipe makes 1½ cups (12 fl oz/375 ml).

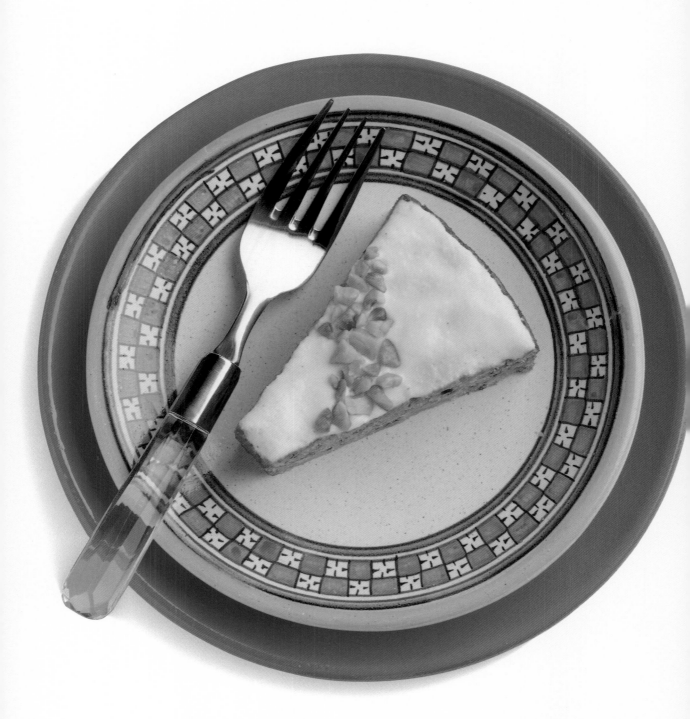

Buttermilk imparts tenderness and bananas richness—plus lots of potassium—to this cake. Beat the eggs for the full time, to help lighten the batter. For a simpler presentation, omit the icing and dust with sifted confectioners' (icing) sugar.

ORANGE WALNUT CAKE

Serves 16

1 egg
¾ cup (6 oz/185 g) sugar
1 cup (4½ oz/140 g) self-rising flour
1 teaspoon baking soda
  (bicarbonate of soda)
1 teaspoon vanilla extract (essence)
grated zest of 1 large orange
½ cup (2 oz/60 g) shelled walnuts,
  toasted and chopped

½ cup (4 fl oz/125 ml) lowfat
  buttermilk
2 very ripe bananas, 8 oz (250 g)
  each, peeled and well mashed
2 tablespoons fresh orange juice
1 cup (8 fl oz/250 ml) Ricotta
  Icing *(recipe on page 124)*
1 tablespoon Grand Marnier

1. Preheat an oven to 350°F (180°C).
2. Coat the inside of a tube pan 9 inches (23 cm) in diameter with nonstick cooking spray.
3. In a bowl, using an electric mixer set on medium speed, beat the egg until foamy, about 2 minutes. Continue to beat, adding the sugar, a few tablespoons at a time, until the mixture is thick and pale yellow, at least 5 minutes. Add the flour, baking soda, vanilla extract, orange zest, half of the toasted nuts, the buttermilk, bananas and orange juice, folding in gently.
4. Spread the batter into the prepared pan. Bake until a toothpick inserted into the center comes out clean, about 30 minutes. Cool completely in the pan, about 10 minutes.
5. Transfer the cooled cake onto a serving plate. In a small bowl, combine the Ricotta Icing and Grand Marnier. Frost the cake with the icing and sprinkle the top with the remaining toasted nuts.
6. To serve, slice into wedges and place on individual plates.

Nutritional Analysis Per Serving:

**CALORIES 138
(KILOJOULES 581)
PROTEIN 4 G
CARBOHYDRATES 23 G
TOTAL FAT 3 G
SATURATED FAT 1 G
CHOLESTEROL 16 MG
SODIUM 208 MG
DIETARY FIBER 1 G**

Even though this cake is made with nonfat sour cream, it tastes surprisingly rich. Arrange the pineapple rings in a pattern that will look attractive on a serving platter. Garnish with edible, non-toxic lemon leaves.

Pineapple Upside-Down Cake

Serves 8

4 tablespoons (2 oz/60 g) unsalted butter, at room temperature

½ cup (3 ½ oz/105 g) firmly packed brown sugar

¼ teaspoon freshly grated nutmeg

¼ cup (2 fl oz/60 ml) water

6 fresh or canned pineapple slices, each ¼ inch (6 mm) thick

¼ cup (2 fl oz/60 ml) nonfat sour cream

¾ cup (6 oz/185 g) granulated sugar

1 egg, beaten

¼ teaspoon coconut flavoring

¾ cup (6 fl oz/180 ml) lowfat milk

1½ cups (7 oz/220 g) self-rising flour

Nutritional Analysis Per Serving:

Calories 304

(Kilojoules 1,278)

Protein 5 g

Carbohydrates 56 g

Total Fat 7 g

Saturated Fat 4 g

Cholesterol 44 mg

Sodium 345 mg

Dietary Fiber 1 g

1. Preheat an oven to 350°F (180°C).

2. In a cast-iron frying pan or a 9-inch (23-cm) cake pan, over medium heat, melt 2 tablespoons of the butter. Add the brown sugar, nutmeg and water to the pan and bring to a boil, stirring to dissolve the sugar. Place the pineapple slices in the butter and cook over medium heat, stirring occasionally, until they are tender and have rendered their juices, 10–15 minutes for fresh, 8–10 minutes for canned.

3. Using a slotted spatula, transfer the pineapple slices to a plate. Cook the juices over medium-high heat until golden, about 5 minutes.

4. Meanwhile, in a food processor fitted with the metal blade, combine the sour cream and granulated sugar. Process until creamy and light, about 5 seconds. Alternatively, in a bowl, using an electric mixer set on medium speed, beat together the sour cream and sugar until creamy and light, about 30 seconds. Using a spatula, stir in the egg and coconut flavoring. Stir to mix well. Then stir in the milk and flour, again mixing well until fully combined.

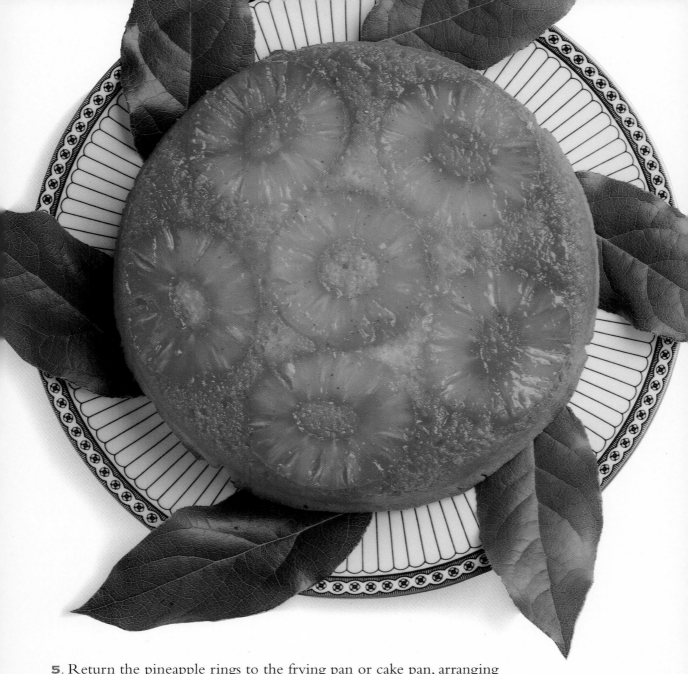

5. Return the pineapple rings to the frying pan or cake pan, arranging them in a single layer. Spoon the batter evenly over the pineapple slices. Bake until golden brown and bubbly, about 30 minutes. Cool completely in the pan, about 20 minutes.

6. To serve, invert a serving plate over the top of the pan and, holding the pan and plate together firmly, invert them. Lift off the pan, allowing any sauce that remains in the bottom to run over the cake.

Containing no egg yolks or other fat, angel food cakes are airy. Because they are leavened by egg whites alone, proper whisking is essential. Use an absolutely clean bowl and room-temperature egg whites. Don't overbeat, or the cake will fall.

CHOCOLATE ANGEL FOOD CAKE

Serves 16

1 cup (4 oz/125 g) cake (soft-wheat) flour, sifted after measuring
¼ cup (1 oz/30 g) plus 2 table-spoons unsweetened cocoa
1¼ cups (10 oz/315 g) granulated sugar

1½ cups egg whites (10–12 whites), at room temperature
1½ teaspoons cream of tartar
1⁄16 teaspoon salt
2 teaspoons vanilla extract (essence)
¼ cup (3 oz/90 g) molasses
2 tablespoons confectioners' (icing) sugar

1. Preheat an oven to 300°F (150°C).
2. In a bowl, sift together the flour, the ¼ cup (1 oz/30 g) cocoa and ½ cup (4 oz/125 g) of the granulated sugar. Set aside.
3. In a large bowl, using an electric mixer set on medium speed or a whisk, beat the egg whites until foamy, about 3 minutes. Add the cream of tartar and salt and continue beating until soft peaks form. With the mixer running, or while constantly beating with the whisk, sprinkle in the remaining ¾ cup (6 oz/180 g) granulated sugar, a little at a time, beating until the egg whites are stiff. Using a rubber spatula, fold in the vanilla extract and molasses. Gently fold the flour mixture into the beaten whites, a little at a time.
4. Carefully spoon the batter into a clean, dry 10-inch (25-cm) angel food cake or other tube pan. Bake until the top springs back when lightly touched and is golden brown, 45–55 minutes. Invert the pan to cool completely, 30–40 minutes.
5. In a small bowl, combine the 2 tablespoons cocoa and confectioners' sugar.
6. To serve, remove the cake from the pan, sieve the cocoa mixture on top, cut into wedges and place on individual plates.

Nutritional Analysis Per Serving:

CALORIES 131
(KILOJOULES 548)
PROTEIN 3 G
CARBOHYDRATES 29 G
TOTAL FAT 0 G
SATURATED FAT 0 G
CHOLESTEROL 0 MG
SODIUM 48 MG
DIETARY FIBER 1 G

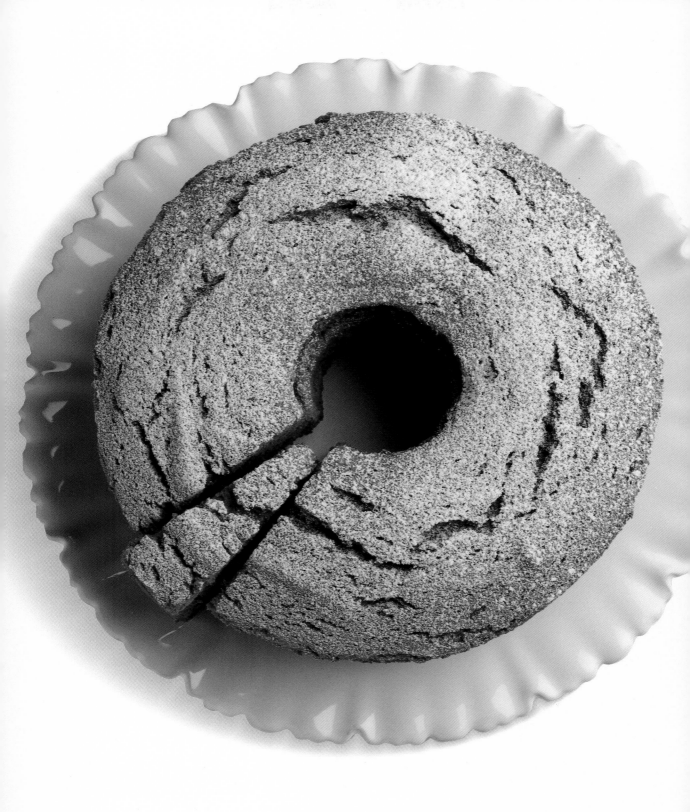

Lowfat and nonfat dairy products replace their richer counterparts in this version of a classic cheesecake. Slow baking and cooling in the oven help prevent the surface from cracking. The finished cheesecake, with topping, will be 1 inch (2.5 cm) high.

Almond Cheesecake

Serves 10

28 vanilla wafers, crumbled
1 egg white, lightly beaten
8 oz (250 g) lowfat cream cheese
2 cups (16 oz/500 g) Yogurt Cheese *(recipe on page 124)* or nonfat sour cream
½ cup (3 ½ oz/105 g) superfine (caster) sugar
1 egg

¼ cup (1½ oz/45 g) all-purpose (plain) flour
1 teaspoon almond extract (essence)
2 tablespoons amaretto liqueur or 1 additional teaspoon almond extract (essence)
½ cup (4 fl oz/125 ml) nonfat sour cream
5 strawberry halves

Nutritional Analysis Per Serving:

Calories 230
(Kilojoules 964)
Protein 9 g
Carbohydrates 31 g
Total Fat 7 g
Saturated Fat 3 g
Cholesterol 35 mg
Sodium 203 mg
Dietary Fiber 0 g

1. Preheat an oven to 325°F (180°C). Coat an 8-inch (20-cm) springform pan with 3-inch (7.5-cm) sides with nonstick cooking spray.

2. In a food processor fitted with the metal blade, combine the wafer crumbs and egg white and pulse just to blend. Transfer the crumb mixture to the prepared pan and press onto the bottom of the pan.

3. In a bowl, using an electric mixer set on medium speed, beat together the cream cheese, Yogurt Cheese or sour cream and sugar until creamy, 2–3 minutes. Add the egg, flour, almond extract and amaretto, if using, and beat to mix completely, 1 minute longer.

4. Spread the filling onto the prepared crust and smooth the top with a rubber spatula. Bake until the center is set, about 1 hour. Turn off the oven and, with the oven door slightly open, cool the cake completely in the oven, about 1 hour longer. Cover the cooled cake and refrigerate until chilled, 2–3 hours.

5. To serve, remove the pan sides. Carefully transfer to a serving plate. Using a spatula, spread the sour cream over the top. Garnish with the strawberry halves. Cut into wedges.

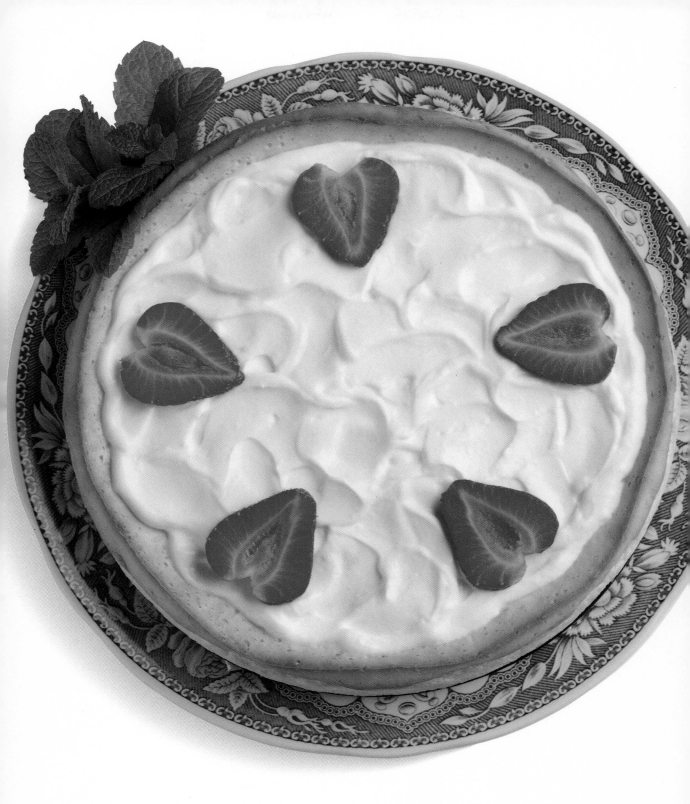

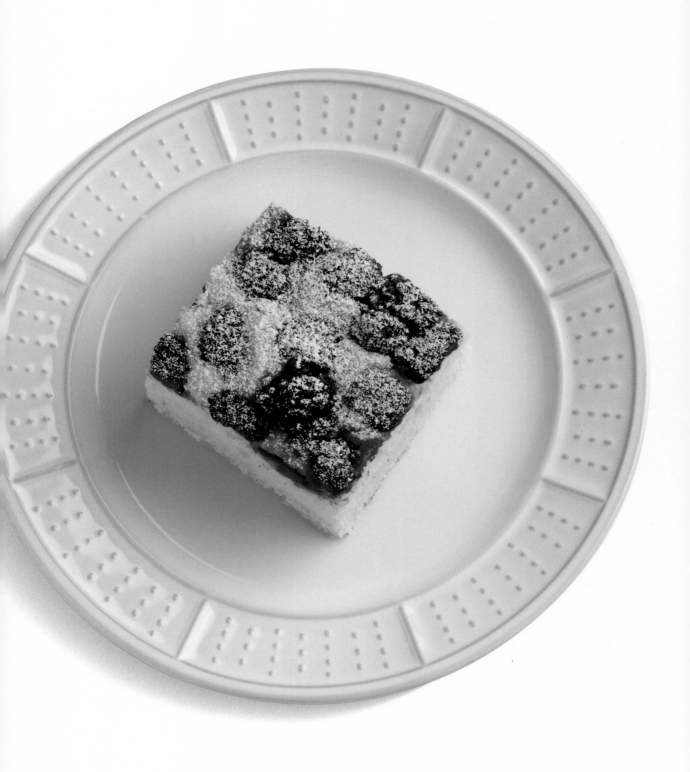

A combination of whole blackberries and sugar creates an appealingly
sticky topping for a cake lightened with nonfat sour cream and lowfat milk.
Whole frozen blackberries can be substituted.

BLACKBERRY CAKE

Serves 9

6 tablespoons (3 oz/90 g) unsalted
  butter
1¼ cups (10 oz/315 g) granulated
  sugar
1 egg
grated zest of ½ lemon
2½ cups (12½ oz/390 g) all-purpose
  (plain) flour

⅟₁₆ teaspoon salt
2 teaspoons baking powder
1½ cups (12 fl oz/375 ml)
  lowfat milk
2 tablespoons nonfat sour cream
2 cups (8 oz/250 g) blackberries
¼ cup (1 oz/30 g) confectioners' (icing)
  sugar, sifted before measuring

1. Preheat an oven to 350°F (180°C). Coat a 9-inch (23-cm)
square baking pan with nonstick cooking spray.
2. In a food processor fitted with the metal blade, combine the
butter and 1 cup (8 oz/250 g) of the granulated sugar. Process
until light and creamy, about 1 minute. Add the egg and pulse a
few times to incorporate fully. Stir in the lemon zest. Alternatively,
place the butter and 1 cup (8 oz/250 g) of the granulated sugar
in a bowl and, using an electric mixer set on medium speed, beat
until light and creamy, about 2 minutes. Beat in the egg until
thoroughly combined and stir in the lemon zest.
3. In a large bowl, combine the flour, salt and baking powder.
Stir the butter mixture into the flour mixture until well combined.
Add the milk and sour cream and stir until the batter is moistened.
4. Spoon the batter into the prepared pan. Spread the blackberries
over the top and then sprinkle evenly with the remaining ¼ cup
(2 oz/60 g) granulated sugar. Bake until a toothpick inserted in
the center comes out clean, about 45 minutes.
5. To serve, sift on the confectioners' sugar, cut into squares and
place on individual plates.

*Nutritional Analysis
Per Serving:*

**CALORIES 374
(KILOJOULES 1,570)
PROTEIN 6 G
CARBOHYDRATES 67 G
TOTAL FAT 10 G
SATURATED FAT 5 G
CHOLESTEROL 48 MG
SODIUM 155 MG
DIETARY FIBER 2 G**

The rich flavor of ripe fruit transforms lowfat cakes and tea breads into satisfying desserts. Here, bananas are used; applesauce would also be good. The riper the bananas, the sweeter the cake will taste, so choose fruit with peels covered in dark brown spots.

Banana Spice Cake

Serves 12

½ cup (4 fl oz/125 ml) vegetable oil
½ teaspoon vanilla extract (essence)
¼ tablespoon nonfat sour cream
½ cup (3½ oz/105 g) firmly packed brown sugar
1 large, very ripe banana, peeled and mashed
1 cup (5 oz/155 g) unbleached all-purpose (plain) flour

1 cup (5 oz/155 g) whole-wheat (wholemeal) flour
2 teaspoons baking powder
1 teaspoon baking soda (bicarbonate of soda)
½ teaspoon ground allspice
1 teaspoon ground cinnamon
2 egg whites
2 tablespoons confectioners' (icing) sugar, sifted before measuring

Nutritional Analysis Per Serving:

CALORIES 214
(KILOJOULES 898)
PROTEIN 4 G
CARBOHYDRATES 30 G
TOTAL FAT 10 G
SATURATED FAT 1 G
CHOLESTEROL 0 MG
SODIUM 200 MG
DIETARY FIBER 2 G

1. Preheat an oven to 350°F (180°C). Coat an 8-inch (20-cm) square cake pan with nonstick cooking spray. Sprinkle lightly with flour, then tap out any excess.

2. In a food processor fitted with the metal blade, combine the vegetable oil, vanilla extract, sour cream and brown sugar. Process until light and creamy, 30–60 seconds. Add the banana and pulse just until incorporated. Alternatively, in a bowl, using an electric mixer set on high speed, beat together the oil, vanilla, sour cream and sugar until creamy and light, 2–3 minutes. Add the banana and beat until incorporated.

3. In a bowl, stir together the all-purpose and whole-wheat flours, baking powder, baking soda, allspice and cinnamon. Stir the creamed mixture into the flour mixture until thoroughly combined.

4. In a clean bowl, using clean beaters, beat the egg whites until stiff peaks form. Using a rubber spatula, fold the beaten whites into the banana mixture.

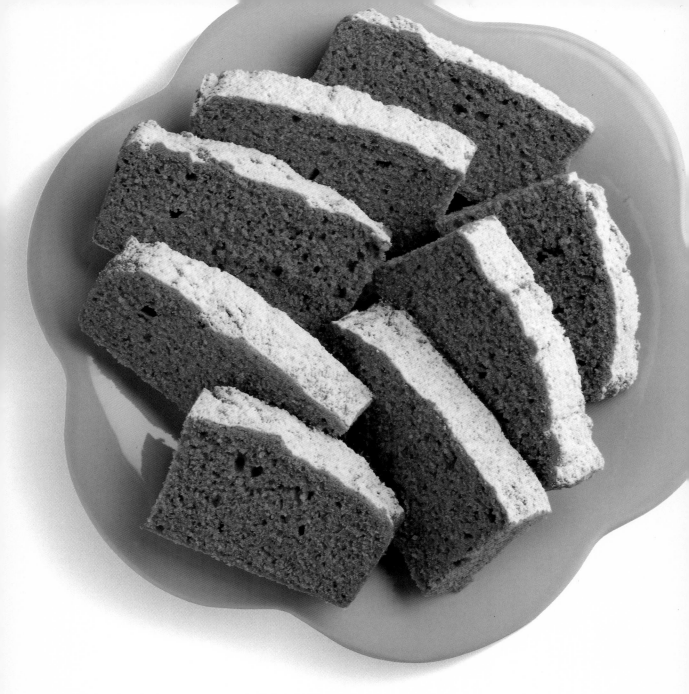

5. Spoon the batter into the prepared dish. Bake until a
toothpick inserted into the center comes out clean, about
45 minutes. Cool completely in the pan, about 20 minutes.
6. To serve, remove from the pan, sift on the confectioners'
sugar, slice and place on a serving platter.

This version of a favorite dessert or teatime loaf comes in at about one-fourth the amount of fat found in most zucchini breads. Yet, it is every bit as delicious—if not more so—with the inclusion of fresh orange juice.

Zucchini & Orange Bread

Serves 12

1½ cups (7½ oz/235 g) whole-wheat (wholemeal) flour

1 cup (8 oz/250 g) sugar

2 teaspoons baking powder

2 eggs, beaten

¼ cup (2 fl oz/60 ml) vegetable oil

2 zucchini (courgettes), grated (2 cups/10 oz/315 g)

¼ cup (2 fl oz/60 ml) fresh orange juice

1. Preheat an oven to 350°F (180°C). Coat a 9-inch (23-cm) loaf pan with nonstick cooking spray.

2. In a bowl, stir together the flour, sugar and baking powder. In another bowl, stir together the eggs, vegetable oil, zucchini and orange juice. Stir the egg mixture into the flour mixture just until moistened. Do not overmix.

3. Spoon the batter into the prepared pan. Bake until the center is firm and the sides are brown and crusty, about 1 hour. Cool in the pan for 10 minutes. Remove from the pan to cool completely, about 20 minutes longer.

4. To serve, cut into slices and place on a serving platter.

Nutritional Analysis Per Serving:

Calories 193

(Kilojoules 811)

Protein 4 g

Carbohydrates 33 g

Total Fat 6 g

Saturated Fat 1 g

Cholesterol 35 mg

Sodium 94 mg

Dietary Fiber 2 g

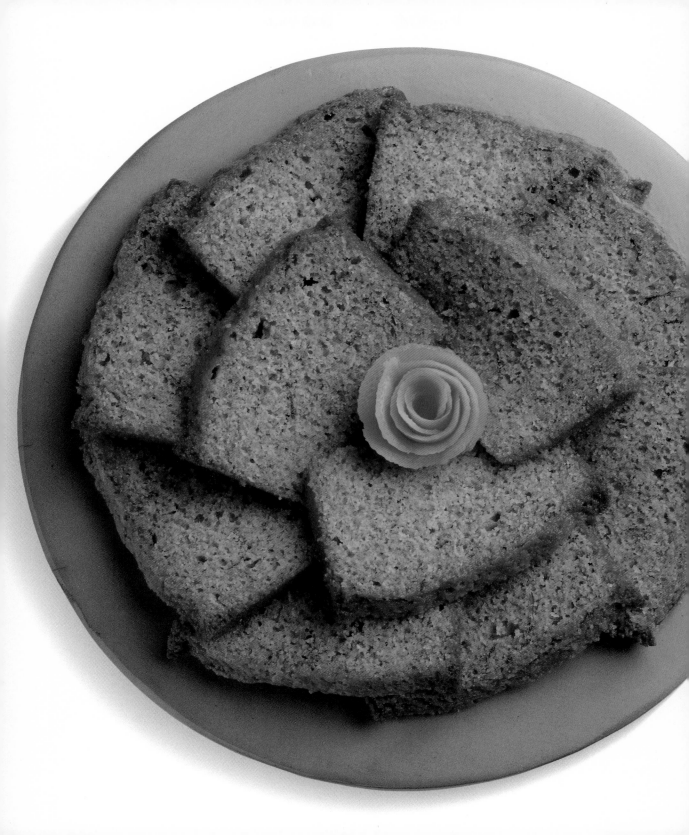

Thin leaves of filo dough, reminiscent of a traditional strudel's richer sheets of pastry, provide a satisfying lowfat option. The filling can be made a few hours in advance of baking and stored in the refrigerator until you are ready to use it.

APPLE STRUDEL

Serves 12

8 apples 1½ lb (750 g) total weight, peeled, quartered, cored and cut into ½-inch (12-mm) pieces
3 tablespoons brown sugar

1 tablespoon fresh lemon juice
1 teaspoon ground allspice
6 filo sheets
2 tablespoons unsalted butter, melted
2 tablespoons confectioners' (icing) sugar

1. Preheat the oven to 350° (180°C).

2. In a large mixing bowl, combine the apples, brown sugar, lemon juice and allspice. Stir to mix well.

3. Lay 2 sheets of the filo dough on a work surface, one directly on top of the other, and brush the sheet on top with one-third of the melted butter. Lay 2 more sheets on top and brush the top sheet again with half of the remaining melted butter.

4. Place the final 2 sheets on top, and then spread the apple mixture over the filo, leaving a 1-inch (2.5-cm) border on all sides. Starting from a long side, tightly roll up the strudel. Press the ends together. Place the roll, seam side down, on a baking sheet. Brush the top with the remaining melted butter.

5. Bake until the top is golden and crisp and the apples are bubbly, 35–40 minutes. Remove from the oven and sift the confectioners' sugar evenly over the top.

6. To serve, cut into slices and place on a serving platter.

Nutritional Analysis Per Serving:

CALORIES 91
(KILOJOULES 384)
PROTEIN 1 G
CARBOHYDRATES 17 G
TOTAL FAT 3 G
SATURATED FAT 1 G
CHOLESTEROL 5 MG
SODIUM 48 MG
DIETARY FIBER 1 G

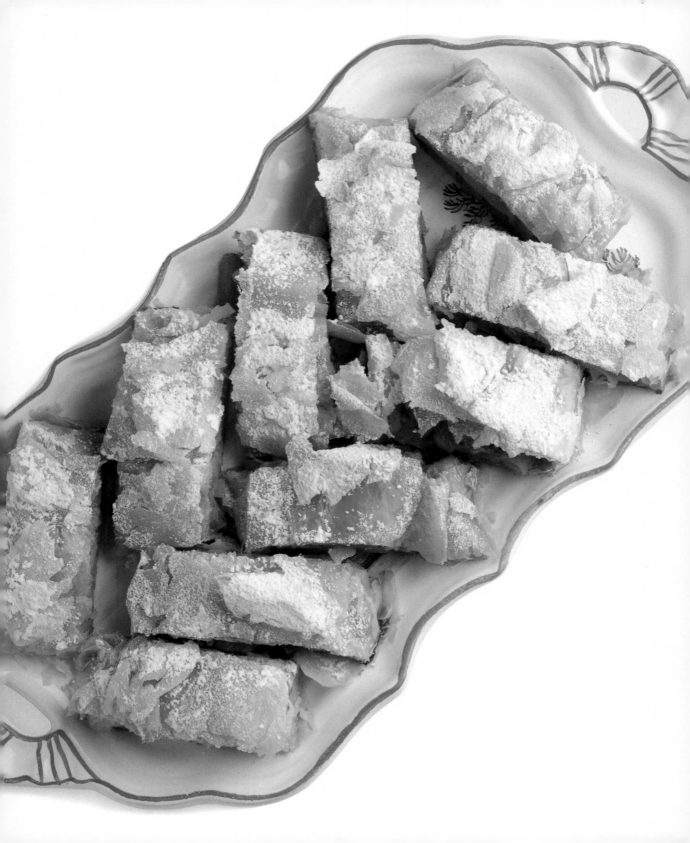

Vanilla Sugar adds extra fragrance to these crisp-surfaced, fluffy waffles. Use fresh or canned sour cherries for the Fruit Coulis, using some more of the chopped cherries scattered into the waffle batter for an intriguing flavor and texture.

SOUR CHERRY WAFFLES

Serves 6

1½ cups (12 fl oz/375 ml) lowfat (1%) milk
2 tablespoons vegetable oil
1 vanilla bean, split in half lengthwise
1½ cups (7½ oz/235 g) all-purpose (plain) flour
1 teaspoon baking powder
¹⁄₁₆ teaspoon salt

¼ cup (2 oz/60 g) Vanilla Sugar *(recipe on page 125)* or granulated sugar
2 tablespoons firmly packed brown sugar
1 whole egg, plus 2 egg whites
½ cup (2½ oz/75 g) chopped, pitted fresh or drained canned sour cherries
Fruit Coulis made with 2 cups (8 oz/ 250 g) pitted fresh or drained canned sour cherries *(recipe on page 125)*

1. Preheat a waffle iron.
2. In a saucepan over medium heat, combine the milk, oil and vanilla bean. When the milk starts to simmer, turn off the heat. Using a sharp knife, scrape the seeds from the vanilla bean halves into the milk, then return the pod halves to the milk. Let the milk cool to room temperature, then discard the bean pods.
3. In a mixing bowl, stir together the flour, baking powder, salt, Vanilla Sugar or granulated sugar and brown sugar. Beat in the cooled milk mixture, the whole egg and the sour cherries.
4. In a clean bowl, using clean beaters, beat the egg whites until stiff peaks form. Using a rubber spatula, fold the beaten egg whites into the flour mixture.
5. Coat the waffle iron with nonstick cooking spray. Spoon ½–¾ cup (4–6 fl oz/125–180 ml) batter onto the hot iron. Close the lid and cook according to the manufacturer's directions; the waffle should be browned and crisp.
6. To serve, place the waffles on individual plates and top with the Fruit Coulis.

Nutritional Analysis Per Serving:

CALORIES 319
(KILOJOULES 1,340)
PROTEIN 8 G
CARBOHYDRATES 56 G
TOTAL FAT 7 G
SATURATED FAT 1 G
CHOLESTEROL 38 MG
SODIUM 167 MG
DIETARY FIBER 1 G

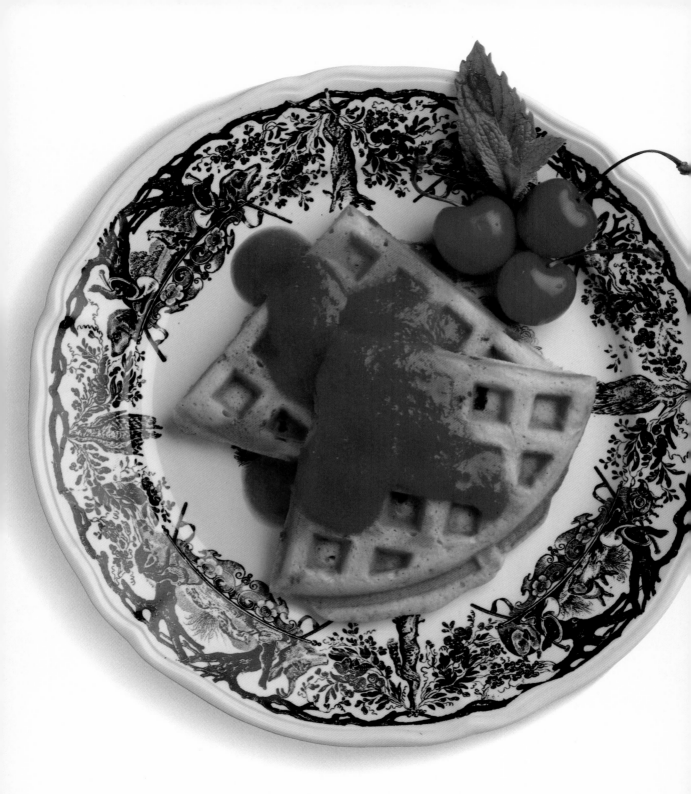

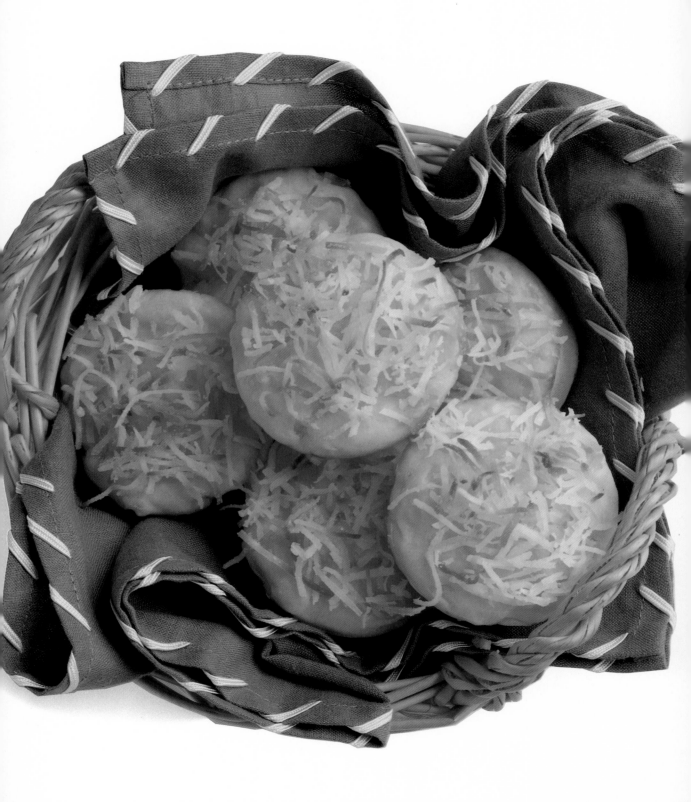

Coconut flavoring adds that popular dessert ingredient's intensely rich taste without any of the fat. Just a small amount of grated coconut is sprinkled on the top of these muffins so its texture can be enjoyed to the fullest.

Pineapple & Coconut Muffins

Makes 6 muffins

1 cup (5 oz/155 g) unbleached
    all-purpose (plain) flour
1 teaspoon baking powder
½ teaspoon baking soda
    (bicarbonate of soda)
1⁄16 teaspoon salt
8 oz (250 g) canned crushed
    pineapple, juice retained

1 egg, separated
1 teaspoon coconut flavoring
    (essence)
1 tablespoon vegetable oil
2 tablespoons firmly packed
    brown sugar
¼ cup (1 oz/30 g) grated
    dried coconut

1. Preheat an oven to 350°F (180°C). Coat the cups of a standard 6-cup muffin tin with nonstick cooking spray.
2. In a medium bowl, stir together the flour, baking powder, baking soda and salt. In a large bowl, combine the pineapple and its juice, the egg yolk, coconut extract, oil and brown sugar. Stir to mix well. Add the flour mixture to the pineapple mixture and stir just until the dry ingredients are moistened.
3. In a clean bowl, using clean beaters, beat the egg white until stiff peaks form. Fold into the flour-pineapple mixture. Do not overmix or tunnels will form in the muffins when they are baked.
4. Spoon the batter into the prepared muffin tin, filling each cup three-fourths full. Bake for 5 minutes. Scatter the grated coconut evenly over the tops and continue to bake until the muffins are golden brown and are beginning to pull away from the sides of the pan, about 30 minutes longer. Cool in the pan for 10 minutes. Turn out of the pan onto a rack to cool completely, about 20 minutes longer.
5. To serve, place in a basket.

*Nutritional Analysis
Per Serving:*

**Calories 184
(Kilojoules 775)
Protein 4 g
Carbohydrates 31 g
Total Fat 5 g
Saturated Fat 2 g
Cholesterol 35 mg
Sodium 233 mg
Dietary Fiber 1 g**

In this typical Eastern European dessert, wholesome buckwheat pancakes enfold a sweet-tart filling of dried apricots—rich in vitamin A, beta-carotene and minerals. Buckwheat flour is very absorbent, so you may have to add water to the batter as it stands.

Buckwheat Crêpes with Apricot Filling

Serves 6

¾ cup (6 fl oz/180 ml) water
¾ cup (6 fl oz/180 ml) lowfat milk
1 egg
⅟₁₆ teaspoon salt
1 teaspoon walnut oil
½ cup (2 oz/60 g) buckwheat flour
½ cup (2½ oz/75 g) all-purpose
   (plain) flour
6 tablespoons (3 oz/90 g) lowfat
   plain yogurt

Apricot Filling

1¼ cups (8 oz/250 g) dried apricots,
   halved
1 cup (8 fl oz/250 ml) hot water
1 large or 2 medium vanilla beans
2 tablespoons fresh orange juice
2 tablespoons sugar
½ teaspoon finely chopped crystallized
   ginger or grated, peeled fresh ginger

1. Prepare the Apricot Filling (see opposite page).
2. In a bowl, whisk together the water, milk, egg, salt and walnut oil. In another bowl, stir together the buckwheat and all-purpose flours. Stir the flour mixture into the liquid mixture until combined; do not overmix. Let the batter stand for 15–20 minutes.
3. Place a 6-inch (15-cm) nonstick frying pan over medium heat. When hot, coat with nonstick cooking spray. Spoon 3 tablespoons of the batter into the pan and tilt the pan to cover the bottom thinly and evenly. Cook until the batter is firm and the edges of the crêpe are starting to become crisp, about 30 seconds. Turn the crêpe out onto a piece of waxed paper. Spray more nonstick cooking spray in the pan and cook the remaining batter in the same way. You should have 12 crêpes in all.
4. To serve, spoon 2 tablespoons Apricot Filling onto the non-browned side of each crêpe. Fold each crêpe in half and then in half again. Place two on each individual plate. Top each with ½ tablespoon of the yogurt.

*Nutritional Analysis
Per Serving:*

Calories 235
(Kilojoules 986)
Protein 7 g
Carbohydrates 48 g
Total Fat 3 g
Saturated Fat 1 g
Cholesterol 39 mg
Sodium 61 mg
Dietary Fiber 4 g

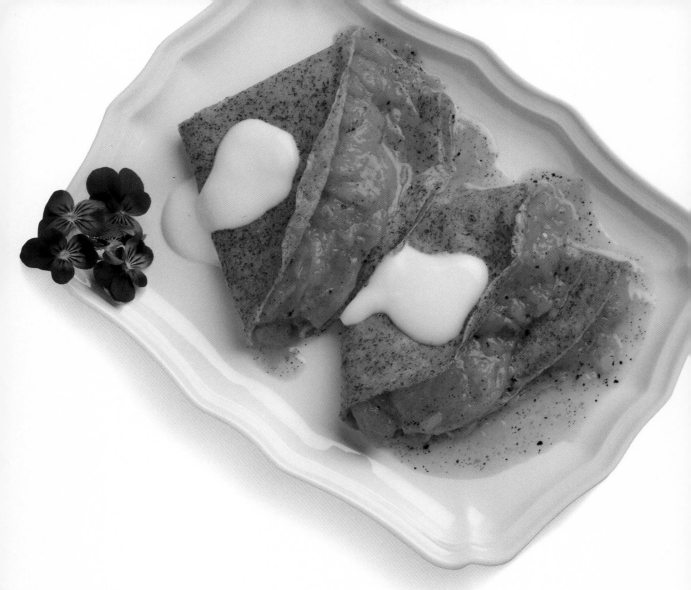

APRICOT FILLING

1. Preheat an oven to 350°F (180°C). Coat a 1-qt (1-l) baking dish with nonstick cooking spray.

2. In a bowl, combine the apricots and water. Let stand until the apricots are plumped, about 10 minutes.

3. Transfer the apricots to the prepared pan. Split the vanilla beans lengthwise and, using the tip of a sharp knife, scrape the seeds onto the apricots. Sprinkle with the orange juice, sugar and ginger and cover the pan with aluminum foil.

4. Bake until the apricots are bubbling and golden, 30–45 minutes. Keep warm until use. This recipe makes 2½ cups (20 oz/625 g).

Satisfyingly wholesome, these dense scones are good served, at teatime or for breakfast, as shown here with cream cheese and apricot fruit spread. You'll find the mixed whole grains—oats, millet, buckwheat, corn and wheat berries—at natural food stores.

Whole-Wheat & Currant Scones

Makes 8 scones

1 cup (5 oz/155 g) unbleached all-purpose (plain) flour

1 cup (5 oz/155 g) whole-wheat (wholemeal) pastry flour

¼ cup (1½ oz/45 g) mixed whole grains

2 teaspoons baking powder

¹⁄₁₆ teaspoon salt

¼ cup (2 oz/60 g) unsalted butter

¼ cup (1½ oz/45 g) dried currants plumped in ¼ cup (2 fl oz/60 ml) apple juice or fresh orange juice

1 egg, lightly beaten

2 tablespoons nonfat sour cream

Nutritional Analysis Per Scone:

Calories 210
(Kilojoules 883)
Protein 6 g
Carbohydrates 32 g
Total Fat 7 g
Saturated Fat 4 g
Cholesterol 42 mg
Sodium 152 mg
Dietary Fiber 3 g

1. Preheat an oven to 400°F (200°C).

2. In a food processor fitted with the metal blade, combine the unbleached flour, whole-wheat flour, mixed grains, baking powder and salt. Process just to combine. Add the butter and pulse a few times until the mixture resembles coarse meal. Add the currants and pulse just until mixed. Add the egg and sour cream and process just until the dough gathers together into a ball. Alternatively, mix together the flours, grains, baking powder and salt in a bowl. Add the butter and, using a pastry blender or your fingers, work together the ingredients until the mixture resembles coarse meal. Stir in the currants and then add the egg and sour cream. Stir and toss with a fork until the mixture comes together into a ball.

3. Turn out the dough onto a floured work surface and knead a few times until smooth. Roll out the dough into a round 1 inch (2.5 cm) thick. Using a round biscuit cutter 2½ inches (6 cm) in diameter, cut out 8 scones. Dip the biscuit cutter into flour between each cut if it begins to stick to the dough. Arrange the scones ½ inch (12 mm) apart on an ungreased baking sheet.

4. Bake until the scones are golden brown, 10–12 minutes. Transfer to a rack to cool, about 5 minutes.

5. To serve, place whole or split on individual plates.

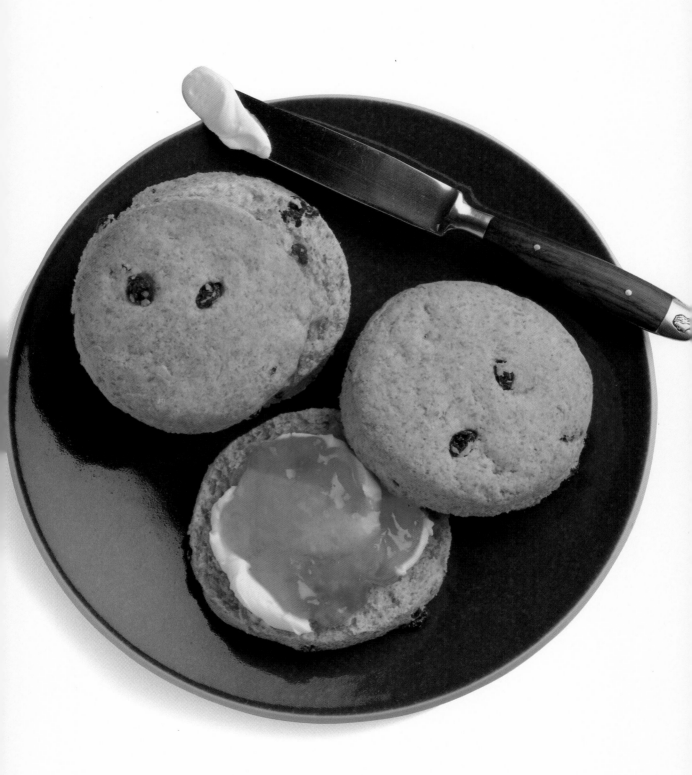

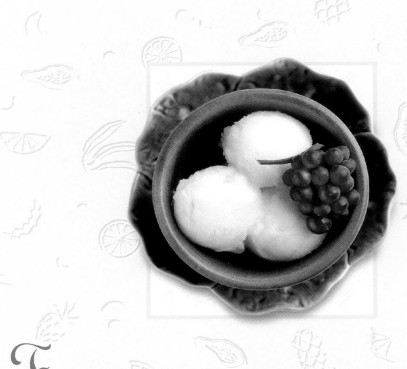

FROZEN CONFECTIONS

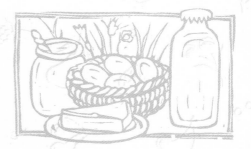

The recipes in this chapter show off the wide range of frozen desserts. The clever use of lowfat dairy products and seasonal fruit for sweetening make for desserts that look good, taste good and are good for you. The frosty fruit slushes, icy sorbets, frothy frozen soufflés and other specialties on the following pages offer chilling satisfaction with far fewer calories than most commercial products. Even the luscious creaminess of old-fashioned ice cream is not lacking. Frozen Vanilla Yogurt and Peaches & Buttermilk Ice prove that there are ways to achieve rich taste and smooth texture without excessive fat. Indeed, these recipes may reshape your personal concept of frozen desserts. While many of them make great, healthy treats for children, others, like Iced Chocolate Bars intensified with a shot of chocolate liqueur, are strictly grown-up delights. Remember that none need be confined to hot summer months, serve them any time you wish to end a meal on a cool, refreshing note.

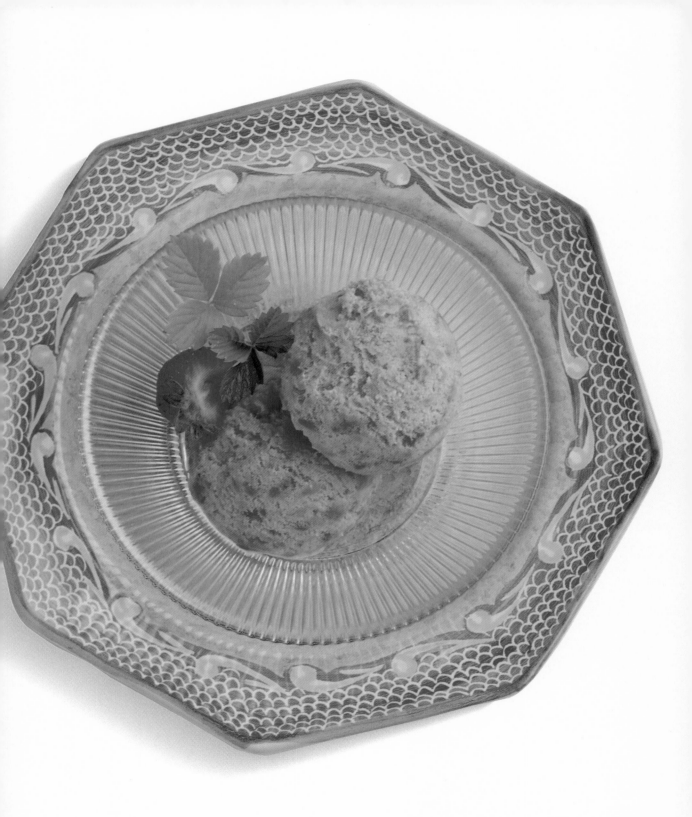

For the best results in this light, frothy dessert, steep the tea until very strong and buy the sweetest strawberries possible. For a special presentation, freeze the mousse in individual soufflé cups and unmold onto individual plates.

STRAWBERRY & LEMON-HIBISCUS TEA MOUSSE

Serves 10

3 cups (12 oz/375 g) ripe strawberries, stems removed and chopped, plus 5 strawberries, stems removed and halved

2 tablespoons crème de framboise liqueur or cranberry juice

⅔ cup (5 oz/155 g) superfine (caster) sugar

¼ cup (2 fl oz/60 ml) brewed lemon-hibiscus tea, chilled

1½ cups (12 oz/375 ml) lowfat milk, placed in the freezer for 1 hour

1. Chill a 2-qt (2-l) bowl.

2. In a food processor fitted with the metal blade, combine the chopped strawberries, liqueur or juice, sugar and chilled tea. Process until just puréed; small bits of strawberry should be visible. Transfer to a large bowl.

3. In a chilled bowl, using chilled beaters, whip the milk until stiff peaks form. If the milk does not whip easily, return it to the freezer for 15 minutes and then whip again. Gently fold the whipped milk into the strawberry mixture. Spoon into the chilled bowl. Cover with plastic wrap, making sure the wrap is set directly against the mousse. Freeze for at least 4 hours or for up to 3 days.

4. To serve, scoop into small bowls and garnish with the strawberry halves.

Nutritional Analysis Per Serving:

**CALORIES 92
(KILOJOULES 387)
PROTEIN 1 G
CARBOHYDRATES 19 G
TOTAL FAT 1 G
SATURATED FAT 0 G
CHOLESTEROL 3 MG
SODIUM 20 MG
DIETARY FIBER 1 G**

A sugar syrup yields a sorbet with a very smooth texture; chill the syrup before adding the Champagne or you'll get rock candy instead. Beaten egg whites, added toward the end of freezing, further lighten the texture.

CHAMPAGNE SORBET

Serves 5

¾ cup (5 oz/155 g) superfine (caster) sugar

1 cup (8 fl oz/250 ml) water

½ cup (4 fl oz/125 ml) citrus-flavored sparkling water

½ cup (4 fl oz/125 ml) Champagne or other sparkling wine

2 egg whites

1. In a heavy saucepan over high heat, combine the sugar and water. Bring to a boil, stirring constantly until the sugar dissolves and the mixture thickens to a syrupy consistency, about 5 minutes. Remove from the heat and let cool to room temperature.

2. Stir in the sparkling water and Champagne or sparkling wine. Pour the mixture into a shallow container, such as an ice cube tray. Place in the freezer and freeze until the mixture turns slushy but is not frozen hard, 30 minutes.

3. Just before the slushy mixture is ready, in a clean bowl, using clean beaters, beat the egg whites until stiff peaks form.

4. Using a fork, break up the slushy mixture. Fold in the beaten egg whites and freeze again until firm, 2–3 hours.

5. To serve, scoop into individual bowls.

Nutritional Analysis Per Serving:

CALORIES 154
(KILOJOULES 648)
PROTEIN 1 G
CARBOHYDRATES 34 G
TOTAL FAT 0 G
SATURATED FAT 0 G
CHOLESTEROL 0 MG
SODIUM 23 MG
DIETARY FIBER 0 G

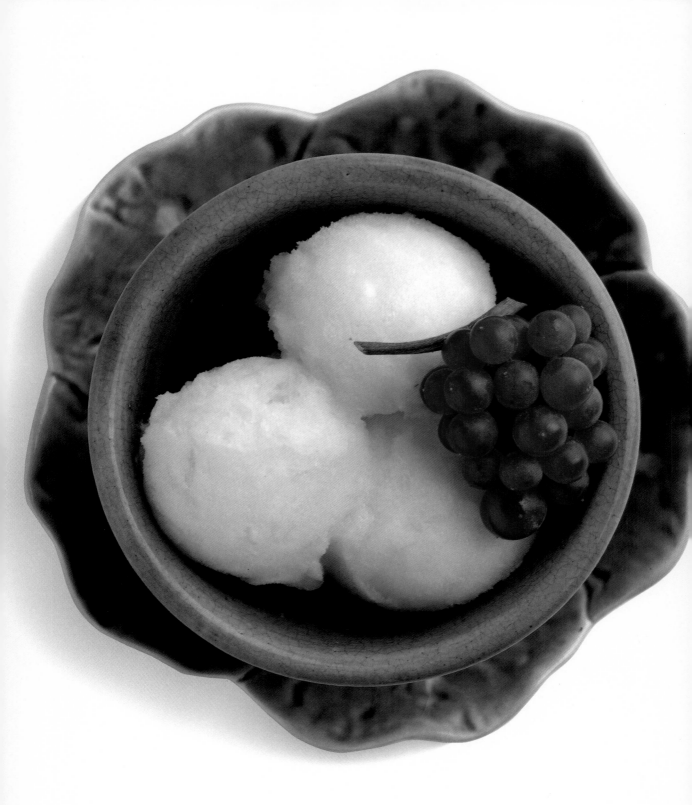

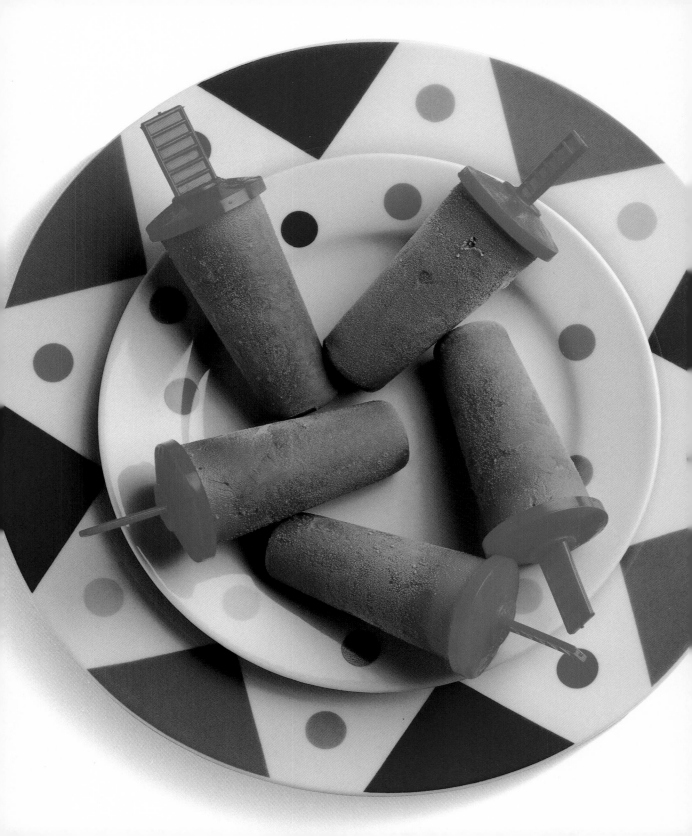

For this grown-up version of a summertime favorite, use a chocolate liqueur with about 34 percent alcohol—low enough to ensure proper freezing. If you'd prefer a smoother dessert, which can be served in bowls, freeze in an ice cream maker.

Iced Chocolate Bars

Makes 8 bars

½ cup (3½ oz/105 g) unsweetened cocoa
½ cup (4 oz/125 g) superfine (caster) sugar
2½ cups (20 fl oz/625 ml) lowfat milk
1 teaspoon vanilla extract (essence)
1 tablespoon chocolate liqueur

1. In a saucepan, stir together the cocoa and sugar. Stir in the milk and place over medium-low heat. Warm, stirring to dissolve the sugar and cocoa, until small bubbles appear along the edge of the pan; do not allow to boil. Remove from the heat.
2. Add the vanilla extract and chocolate liqueur. Stir to mix well.
3. Pour the mixture into ice pop containers with sticks in place. Freeze until frozen hard, about 4 hours.

Nutritional Analysis Per Serving:

**Calories 112
(Kilojoules 471)
Protein 4 g
Carbohydrates 21 g
Total Fat 2 g
Saturated Fat 1 g
Cholesterol 6 mg
Sodium 39 mg
Dietary Fiber 2 g**

Buttermilk gives this confection a velvety texture that belies its low fat content, yielding a combination as appealing to eat as peaches and cream can be. Garnish with fresh peaches. When fresh peaches are out of season, substitute canned ones.

PEACHES & BUTTERMILK ICE

Serves 8

1½ cups (12 fl oz/375 ml) lowfat buttermilk

1 egg

1 cup (8 oz/250 g) Vanilla Sugar *(recipe on page 125)* or granulated sugar

1½ cups (12 fl oz/375 ml) lowfat milk, placed in the freezer for 1 hour

4 peaches, 1¼ lb (625 g) total weight, peeled, halved, pitted and diced

½ teaspoon almond extract (essence)

¹⁄₁₆ teaspoon ground cloves

1. In a saucepan over medium-low heat, warm the buttermilk until just warm.

2. In a bowl, using an electric mixer on medium speed, beat together the egg and Vanilla Sugar or granulted sugar until very pale and frothy, about 3 minutes. Add the egg mixture to the buttermilk and place over medium-low heat. Warm the mixture, stirring continually, for 5 minutes; do not allow it to boil. Cool to room temperature.

3. In a chilled bowl, using chilled beaters, whip the milk until soft peaks form. If the milk does not whip easily, return it to the freezer for 15 minutes and then whip again. Fold the whipped milk into the cooled egg-buttermilk mixture and add the peaches. Add the almond extract and cloves and stir to mix well.

4. Pour the mixture into a shallow pan, such as a cake pan, and freeze until solid, about 4 hours. Alternatively, pour the mixture into an ice cream maker and freeze according to the manufacturer's instructions.

5. To serve, scoop into individual bowls.

Nutritional Analysis Per Serving:

CALORIES 185
(KILOJOULES 777)
PROTEIN 4 G
CARBOHYDRATES 39 G
TOTAL FAT 2 G
SATURATED FAT 1 G
CHOLESTEROL 32 MG
SODIUM 79 MG
DIETARY FIBER 1 G

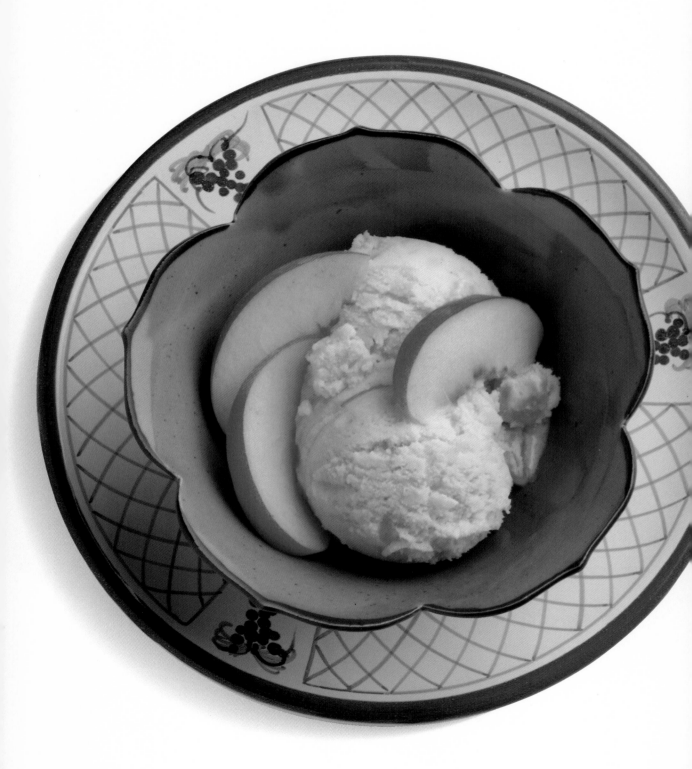

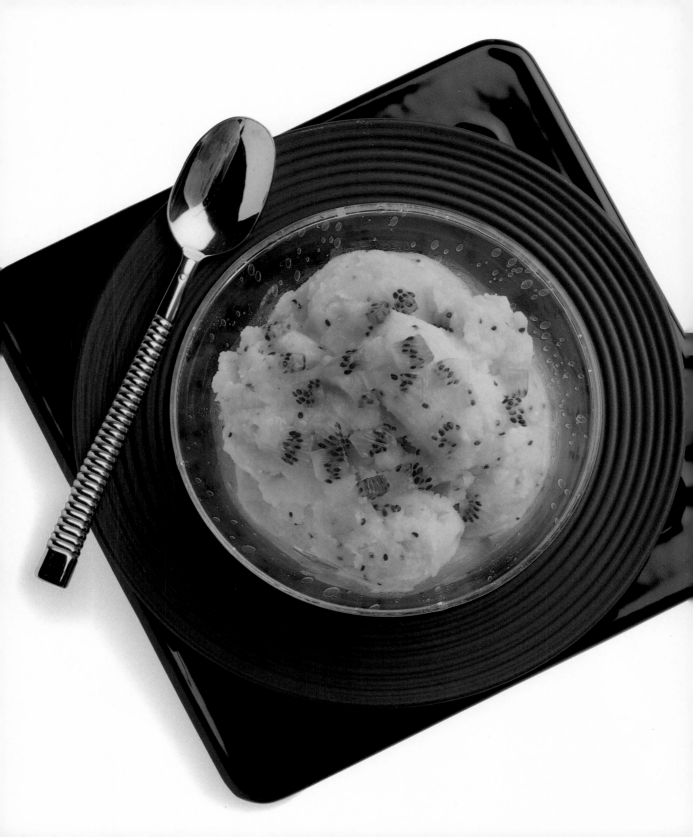

Fresh fruits in season make delightful softened ices, commonly known as slushes. Here, kiwifruit and banana are combined, but feel free to experiment with other fruits such as raspberries, peaches, nectarines, pears or strawberries.

Frozen Fruit Slush

Serves 6

½ cup (4 oz/125 g) Vanilla Sugar *(recipe on page 125)* or granulated sugar
1 cup (8 fl oz/250 ml) water

2 large ripe kiwifruits, 6 oz (185 g) total weight, peeled and sliced
1 large ripe banana, peeled and mashed
2 tablespoons ginger marmalade

1. In a saucepan over high heat, combine the Vanilla Sugar or granulated sugar and water. Bring to a boil, stirring constantly until the sugar dissolves and the mixture thickens to a syrupy consistency, about 5 minutes. Remove from the heat and let cool completely to room temperature.
2. Reserve 6 kiwifruit slices for garnish. Stir the remaining kiwifruits, banana and ginger marmalade into the sugar syrup. Cover and let stand for 1 minute.
3. Transfer to a food processor fitted with the metal blade and purée until smooth.
4. Pour the fruit mixture into a shallow bowl and freeze just long enough for it to become slushy, 30 minutes. Using a fork, break up the mixture. Alternatively, pour the mixture into an ice cream maker and freeze according to the manufacturer's instructions until slushy.
5. To serve, scoop into individual bowls. Cut the reserved kiwi slices into small cubes and scatter an equal amount over the top of each serving.

Nutritional Analysis Per Serving:

CALORIES 125
(KILOJOULES 524)
PROTEIN 0 G
CARBOHYDRATES 32 G
TOTAL FAT 0 G
SATURATED FAT 0 G
CHOLESTEROL 0 MG
SODIUM 5 MG
DIETARY FIBER 1 G

Specks of vanilla bean contribute to the look as well as the flavor of this adult version of frozen yogurt. You can, of course, change the topping to vary the recipe. A beaten egg white keeps the yogurt from becoming too hard to scoop.

Frozen Vanilla Yogurt

Serves 6

3 cups (1½ lb/750 g) nonfat plain yogurt
1 teaspoon vanilla extract (essence)
½ cup (2 oz/60 g) confectioners' (icing) sugar
1 vanilla bean
1 egg white
3 tablespoons scotch whisky
2 teaspoons finely ground espresso roast coffee

1. In a large bowl, stir together the yogurt, vanilla extract and confectioners' sugar. Split the vanilla bean lengthwise and, using the tip of a sharp knife, scrape the seeds into the bowl. Stir to mix well.

2. In a clean bowl, using clean beaters, beat the egg white until stiff peaks form. Gently fold the beaten egg white into the yogurt mixture.

3. Pour the mixture into a shallow pan, such as a cake pan, and freeze until solid, about 4 hours. Alternatively, pour the mixture into an ice cream maker and freeze according to the manufacturer's instructions.

4. To serve, scoop into individual bowls. Spoon 2 teaspoons of the scotch over each serving and sprinkle with an equal amount of the ground coffee.

Nutritional Analysis Per Serving:

CALORIES 124
(KILOJOULES 522)
PROTEIN 7 G
CARBOHYDRATES 19 G
TOTAL FAT 0 G
SATURATED FAT 0 G
CHOLESTEROL 2 MG
SODIUM 96 MG
DIETARY FIBER 0 G

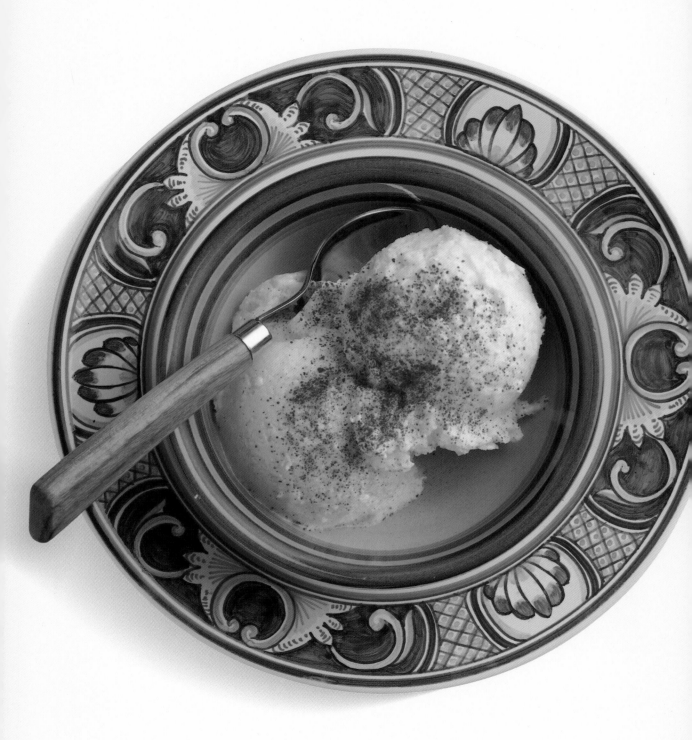

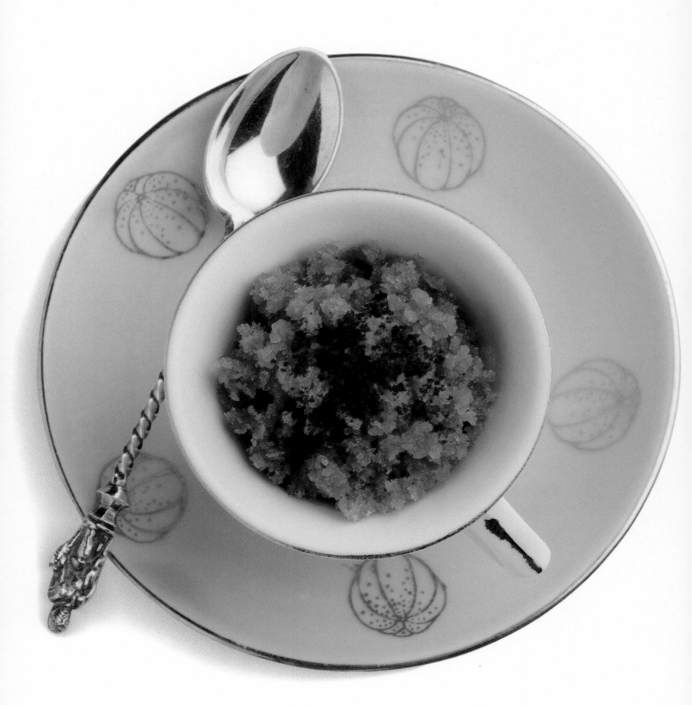

The word *granita* aptly describes the appealingly grainy texture of this icy dessert, which highlights the flavor of good freshly brewed coffee. To achieve the correct consistency, allow ample time for freezing, thawing and refreezing the mixture.

COFFEE GRANITA

Serves 8

3 cups (24 fl oz/750 ml) brewed espresso or double-strength dark-roast coffee

1 cup (8 fl oz/250 ml) lowfat milk

1¼ cups (10 oz/315 g) Vanilla Sugar *(recipe on page 125)* or granulated sugar

4 teaspoons finely ground espresso roast coffee

1. In a saucepan over medium heat, stir together the brewed coffee, milk and Vanilla Sugar or granulated sugar until the mixture almost comes to a boil and the sugar dissolves. Remove from the heat.

2. Pour the mixture into a shallow pan, such as a cake pan, and let cool to room temperature. Place in the freezer to freeze solid, for 3–6 hours.

3. Forty-five minutes before serving, remove from the freezer and thaw for 15 minutes. Using a fork, break up the mixture. Stir to mix well and return to the freezer for 30 minutes.

4. To serve, scoop servings into cups and dust each with ½ teaspoon of the ground coffee.

Nutritional Analysis Per Serving:

CALORIES 157
(KILOJOULES 658)
PROTEIN 1 G
CARBOHYDRATES 38 G
TOTAL FAT 1 G
SATURATED FAT 0 G
CHOLESTEROL 2 MG
SODIUM 19 MG
DIETARY FIBER 0 G

Surprisingly, lowfat milk can be whipped as stiff as whipping cream, provided the milk, bowl and beaters are very cold to begin with. Use a zesting tool to produce long, thin strands of lime zest as a garnish for this intensely flavored frozen soufflé.

FROZEN LIME SOUFFLÉ

Serves 6

¼ cup (2 fl oz/60 ml) water
1 envelope (1 tablespoon) unflavored gelatin
¾ cup (6 fl oz/180 ml) lime juice
½ cup (4 oz/125 g) sugar
grated zest of 2 limes
1½ cups (12 oz/375 ml) lowfat milk, placed in the freezer for 1 hour

1. Coat six ½-cup (4 fl-oz/125-ml) soufflé dishes or molds with nonstick cooking spray. Cut pieces of waxed paper long enough to encircle each dish, then fold each piece to create a strip about 3 inches (7.5 cm) wide. Ring the top of each dish with a strip so that it stands about 2 inches (5 cm) above the rim and tape it in place. Chill the dishes.

2. In a small saucepan, place the water and sprinkle the gelatin over the top. Let stand for 5 minutes to soften. Stir in the lime juice, sugar and half of the lime zest. Place over medium-low heat and stir to dissolve the sugar and gelatin, 3–4 minutes. Remove from the heat and transfer to a large bowl. Let cool until thickened.

3. In a chilled bowl, using chilled beaters, whip the milk until stiff peaks form. If the milk does not whip easily, return it to the freezer for 15 minutes and then whip again. Gently fold the whipped milk into the lime mixture. Divide the mixture evenly among the prepared dishes, spooning it in gently. Freeze the mousse for at least 4 hours or for up to 2 days.

4. To serve, remove the waxed paper from each soufflé dish and set on an individual plate. Garnish with the remaining lime zest.

Nutritional Analysis Per Serving:

CALORIES 117
(KILOJOULES 492)
PROTEIN 3 G
CARBOHYDRATES 24 G
TOTAL FAT 2 G
SATURATED FAT 1 G
CHOLESTEROL 5 MG
SODIUM 38 MG
DIETARY FIBER 0 G

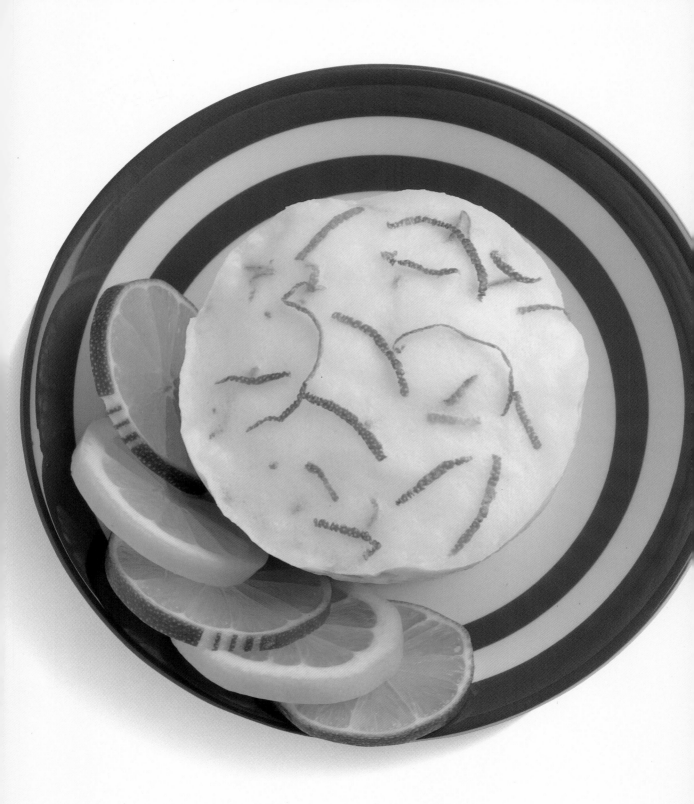

BASIC TERMS & TECHNIQUES

The following entries provide a reference source for this volume, offering definitions of essential or unusual ingredients and explanations of fundamental techniques, geared toward a healthy way of cooking.

BAKING POWDER & BAKING SODA

Commercial baking powder combines baking soda, the source of the carbon dioxide gas that causes quick batters and doughs to rise; an acid, such as cream of tartar, calcium acid phosphate or sodium aluminum sulfate, which, when the powder is combined with a liquid, causes the baking soda to release its gas; and a starch such as cornstarch or flour, to keep the powder from absorbing moisture. Baking soda, also known as bicarbonate of soda or sodium bicarbonate, is often used on its own to leaven batters that include acidic ingredients such as buttermilk, yogurt or citrus juices.

BERRIES

A wide variety of cultivated berries add bright contrasts of color, flavor and texture to desserts, as well as contributing complex carbohydrates, minerals, vitamins A and C and beta-carotene. Usually sold in small containers or baskets, berries should be checked carefully to make sure that they are firm, plump and free of blemishes, bruises or mold. Among berry varieties most widely available are:

BLACKBERRIES Juicy, lustrous purple-black berries, at peak of season in summer.

BLUEBERRIES Small, round berries with smooth, dark-blue skins, available from late spring through summer. Frozen blueberries, available in food stores year-round, are acceptable substitutes for cooked desserts.

CRANBERRIES Round, deep red, tart berries, grown primarily in wet, sandy coastal lands called bogs in the northeastern United States. Available fresh from autumn through early winter and frozen year-round.

LOGANBERRIES These hybrids of the blackberry and raspberry, developed in California and grown throughout the United States, resemble long, shiny raspberries, with a somewhat sharper flavor. Available early to mid-summer.

RASPBERRIES Sweet, small, red berries with a delicate flavor and tender texture. In peak of season during summer, they are also available frozen year-round for use in cooked desserts.

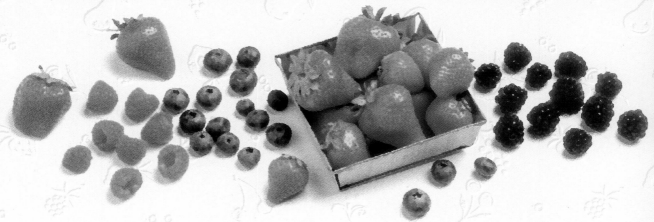

STRAWBERRIES Probably the most popular berry variety, these plump and juicy, intensely sweet, red, heart-shaped fruits are at their peak from spring into mid-summer. Stem or hull strawberries only after washing them, to avoid washing away their sweet juices and spoiling their texture; use a strawberry huller, or the tip of a small, sharp knife, to remove the stem, hull and hard white core of the berry.

BUTTER

The recipes in this book were formulated and analyzed using unsalted butter. Lacking salt, it allows the cook greater leeway in seasoning recipes to taste or to dietary needs.

CHOCOLATE & COCOA

Although chocolate is very high in fat, a small amount goes a long way to add flavor to desserts. Cocoa powder, from which much of the cocoa butter has been removed, provides rich chocolate flavor without adding significant quantities of fat. Purchase the best-quality chocolate you can find—unsweetened, bittersweet, semisweet or sweet, as the recipe requires.

To Chop Chocolate: While a food processor fitted with the metal blade can be used, a sharp, heavy knife offers better control. Break the chocolate by hand into small chunks, handling it as little as possible to avoid melting. Using a heavy knife and a clean, dry, odor-free chopping surface, carefully chop into smaller pieces. Steadying the knife with your hand, continue chopping across the pieces until the desired consistency is reached.

To Melt Chocolate: Put pieces of chocolate in the top pan of a double boiler over barely simmering water, taking care that the pan doesn't touch the water or that the water does not create steam. Stir gently until the chocolate has melted. Alternatively, create your own double boiler by placing a heatproof bowl on top of a pan of simmering water.

CITRUS ZESTS

The thin outermost layer of a citrus fruit's peel, the zest contains most of its aromatic essential oils and remarkable amounts of vitamin C. Zests are a lively source of flavor and make an attractive garnish.

To Zest Citrus Fruit: Using a simple tool known as a zester or a fine handheld shredder, drawing the sharp-edged holes across the fruit's skin, remove the zest in thin strips. Alternatively, holding the edge of a paring knife or vegetable peeler away from you and almost parallel to the fruit's skin, carefully cut off the zest in thin strips, taking care not to remove any white pith with it. Then slice or chop thinly.

EGGS

Eggs are sold in the United States in a range of standard sizes, the most common being jumbo, extra large, large and medium. The recipes in this book were designed for large eggs. While many diet-conscious eaters avoid eggs for their high fat and cholesterol content, egg whites alone are free of both fat and cholesterol and may be used to add body and protein to desserts.

To Separate an Egg: Crack the shell in half by tapping it against the side of a bowl and then breaking it apart with your fingers. Holding the shell halves over the bowl, gently transfer the whole yolk back and forth between them, letting the clear white drop away into the bowl. Take care not to cut into the yolk with the edges of the shell (the whites will not beat properly if they contain any yolk). Transfer the yolk to another bowl. Alternatively, gently pour the egg from the shell onto the slightly cupped fingers of your outstretched clean hand, held over a bowl. Let the whites fall between your fingers into the bowl; the whole yolk will remain in your hand. The same basic function is also performed by an aluminum, ceramic or plastic egg separator placed over a bowl. The separator holds the yolk intact in its cuplike center while allowing the white to drip out through one or more slots in its side into the bowl.

To Whisk Egg Whites: Through a harmless chemical reaction, egg whites adhere to an un-lined half-sphere copper bowl, allowing more air to be beaten into them to achieve a greater and more stable volume. If you don't have a copper bowl, a little cream of tartar added to the whites will also stabilize them, although it will not in-crease their volume.

Put the whites into a large clean bowl. Using a wire whisk or an electric beater set on medium speed, beat the whites with broad, sweeping strokes to incorporate as much air as possible. As the whites begin to thicken and turn a glossy, snowy white, lift out the whisk or beater: If a peak forms and then droops back on itself, the whites have reached the "soft peak" stage. For "stiff peak" whites, continue beating until the whites form stiff, unmoving peaks when the whisk or beater is lifted out.

EXTRACTS

Extracts (essence) are flavorings derived by dissolv-ing essential oils of richly flavored foods—almonds, maple, peppermint, vanilla—in an alco-hol base. Use products labeled "pure" or "natural."

FLOURS

A wide variety of flours may be used in healthy desserts to yield a range of tastes and textures.

ALL-PURPOSE FLOUR The most common flour for general baking is all-purpose flour (also called plain flour), a blend of hard and soft wheats avail-able in all food markets. All-purpose flour is sold in its natural, pale yellow unbleached form or bleached, the result of a chemical process that not only whitens it but also makes it easier to blend with higher percentages of fat and sugar. Bleached flour is therefore commonly used for recipes where more tender results are desired, while unbleached flour yields more crisp results.

BUCKWHEAT FLOUR Ground from the seeds of an herbaceous plant originating in Asia, buckwheat flour is popular in the cuisines of Russia and East-ern Europe. Its strong, earthy, slightly sour flavor is usually modulated in commercial products by the addition of a little whole-wheat flour.

CAKE FLOUR This very fine-textured, low-protein, bleached flour is used in cakes and other baked goods. Also called soft-wheat flour. All-purpose (plain) flour is not an acceptable substitute for cake flour.

SELF-RISING FLOUR A blend of hard and soft wheat flours similar to all-purpose flour, with which baking powder has been combined to make a product that provides its own leavening.

WHOLE-WHEAT FLOUR This pale brown flour, also known as wholemeal or whole-grain flour, is derived from whole, unbleached wheat ber-ries, from which neither the bran nor the germ has been removed; it is thus higher in fiber and minerals than all-purpose or cake flour.

FRUIT SPREADS

Food stores carry naturally sweetened fruit spreads in ever-increasing numbers. Unlike jams, jellies or other commercial preserves, such spreads are made by reducing puréed fruit alone, without sugar, to a thick, spreadable consistency. Fruit juice concentrates usually provide added sweet-ness to the spread.

HERBS

Though herbs are most frequently thought of as a seasoning for savory foods, many have sweet flavors that may also be used to highlight healthy desserts and are particularly complementary to fruits. The various members of the mint family, including peppermint and spearmint, have a brisk, refreshing quality that adds satisfaction without adding calories in any significant numbers.

HONEY

The natural, sweet, syruplike substance produced by bees from flower nectar, honey subtly reflects the color, taste and aroma of the blossoms from which it was made, providing a distinctive mellow sweetness in desserts. Although its health benefits have long been touted, and its flavor is wonderfully wholesome, honey, in fact, does not offer any significant nutritional advantages over sugar. Milder varieties, such as clover and orange blossom, are lighter in color and better suited to general cooking purposes. When substituting honey for sugar in a recipe, reduce other liquids by ¼ cup (2 fl oz/60 ml) for every 1 cup (12 oz/375 g) of honey used, to compensate for the honey's higher moisture content, and reduce baking temperature by 25°F (15°C) to prevent burning.

MAPLE SYRUP

Syrup made from boiling the sap of the maple tree, with an inimitably rich savor and intense sweetness. Buy maple syrup that is labeled "pure," rather than a blend.

MOLASSES

The thick, robust-tasting, syrupy by-product of sugar refining, light molasses results from the first boiling of the syrup; dark molasses from the second boiling; and dark, bitter blackstrap molasses from the third boiling. Blackstrap molasses, considered a health food, has more than four times the calcium, almost four times the iron and over 50 percent more potassium than regular molasses.

NONSTICK COOKING SPRAY

An aerosol mixture of oil, lecithin (a soybean extract used as an emulsifier), sometimes grain alcohol, and a harmless propellant, nonstick cooking sprays allow a fine mist of oil to be applied to a cooking surface thus preventing food from sticking and enabling you to bake or sauté with little added fat.

NUTS

Although nuts are high in fat and should be avoided in large quantities in a healthy diet, they can nevertheless be added to recipes in small quantities to contribute their characteristic flavor and texture—as well as many hard-to-get vitamins and minerals—with little added fat. Toast and chop unsalted shelled nuts at home for the freshest flavor without added fat or salt.

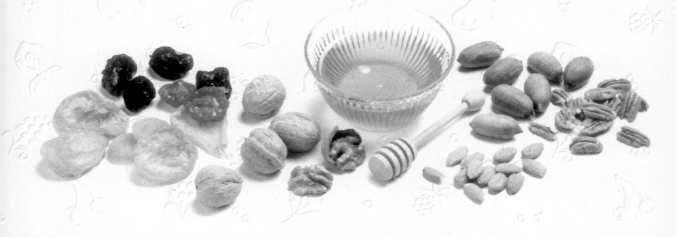

To Toast Nuts: Toasting brings out the full flavor and aroma of nuts. To toast any kind of nut, preheat an oven to 325°F (165°C). Spread the nuts in a single layer on a baking sheet and toast in the oven until they just begin to change color, 5–10 minutes. Remove from the oven and let cool to room temperature. Alternatively, a small quantity of nuts may be toasted in a single layer in a dry heavy frying pan over low heat, stirring frequently to prevent scorching.

To Chop Nuts: Spread them in a single layer on a nonslip cutting surface. Using a chef's knife, carefully chop the nuts with a gentle rocking motion. Alternatively, put a handful or two of nuts in a food processor fitted with the metal blade and use rapid on-off pulses to chop the nuts to desired consistency; repeat with the remaining nuts in batches. Be careful not to process the nuts too long or their oils will be released and the nuts will turn into a paste.

OILS

Although oil is nothing more than a vegetable fat that is liquid at room temperature, and therefore derives 100 percent of its calories from fat, a relatively small amount of oil aids cooking and adds distinctive flavor. Oils are also an excellent source of vitamin E and play an essential role in transporting the fat-soluble vitamins in our diet. Vegetable oils contain no cholesterol. Store all oils in tightly covered containers away from heat and light.

For most dessert-making purposes, use flavorless vegetable and seed oils such as safflower, corn and canola (rapeseed) oil for their high cooking temperatures and bland flavors. Walnut oil is sometimes used in desserts to convey the rich taste of the nuts from which it is pressed; seek out oil made from lightly toasted nuts, which has a full but not too assertive flavor.

SPICES

A wide variety of dried spices—derived from aromatic seeds, roots and barks—enhance the flavor of healthy desserts. As their flavor dissipates quickly, buy spices in relatively small quantities and store them in tightly covered containers away from heat and light. Some of the most common spices, used in this book, include:

ALLSPICE Sweet spice of Caribbean origin with a flavor suggesting a blend of cinnamon, cloves and nutmeg, hence its name. May be purchased as whole dried berries or ground. When using whole berries, first bruise—then gently crushed with the bottom of a pan or other heavy instrument—to release more of their flavor.

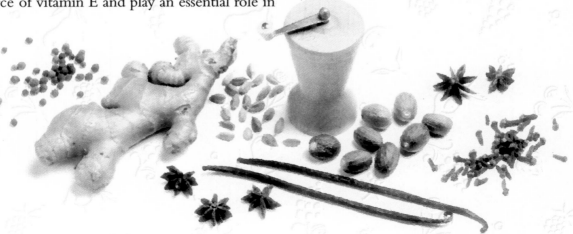

ANISEED A sweet licorice-flavored spice of Mediterranean origin, the small crescent-shaped seeds are related to parsley. Often sold as whole seeds to be crushed with a mortar and pestle.

CARDAMOM This sweet, exotic-tasting spice is used in Middle Eastern and Indian cooking and in Scandinavian baking. Its small, round seeds, which come enclosed inside a husklike pod, are best purchased whole, then ground with a spice grinder or with a mortar and pestle as needed.

CINNAMON A popular sweet spice for flavoring baked goods, cinnamon is the aromatic bark of a type of evergreen tree. It is sold as whole dried strips—cinnamon sticks—or ground.

CLOVES A rich and aromatic East African spice used whole or ground to flavor both sweet and savory recipes.

GINGER The rhizome of the tropical ginger plant yield a sweet, strong-flavored spice. Whole ginger rhizomes, commonly but mistakenly called roots, may be purchased fresh in a food store or vegetable market. Ginger pieces are available crystallized or candied in specialty-food shops or the baking or Asian sections of well-stocked food stores. Ginger preserved in syrup is sold in specialty shops or in Asian food sections. Ground, dried ginger is easily found in jars or tins in the spice section.

NUTMEG This popular baking spice is the hard pit of the fruit of the nutmeg tree. Purchase ground or, for fresher flavor, whole. Whole nutmegs may be kept inside special nutmeg graters, which include hinged flaps that conceal a storage compartment. Freshly grate nutmeg as needed, steadying one end of grater on work surface. Return unused portion of whole nutmeg to the compartment.

STAR ANISE A small, hard, brown seedpod resembling an eight-pointed star, star anise is used whole or broken into individual points to lend its distinctive anise flavor to sweet or savory dishes. The spokes of the star contain small seeds.

VANILLA The dried aromatic pods of a variety of orchid, vanilla beans are a popular flavoring. Vanilla is also commonly used in the form of an alcohol-based extract (essence); be sure to purchase products labeled "pure vanilla extract."

SUGARS

Many different forms of sugar may be used to sweeten desserts.

BROWN SUGAR A rich-tasting granulated sugar combined with molasses in varying quantities to yield golden, light or dark brown sugar, with crystals varying from coarse to finely granulated.

CONFECTIONERS' SUGAR This finely pulverized sugar, also known as powdered or icing sugar, dissolves quickly and provides a thin decorative coating. To prevent confectioners' sugar from absorbing moisture in the air and caking, manufacturers often mix a little cornstarch into it.

GRANULATED SUGAR The standard, widely used form of pure white sugar. Granulated sugar ground to form extra-fine granules is called superfine or castor sugar. Because it dissolves quickly in liquids, it is ideal for some baking recipes. Do not use superfine granulated sugar unless specified.

WINES

Used as flavorings or featured ingredients in fruit salads, ices and some baked goods, still, sparkling and fortified wines add great flavor to healthy desserts. Note: Heat must be applied to wine for about one-half hour for its alcohol content to fully evaporate.

CHAMPAGNE Only French sparkling wine from the Champagne region, made from Chardonnay grapes and noted for its fine bubbles and dry-but-fruity flavor is Champagne. Other sparkling wines may be substituted.

BASIC RECIPES

The following basic recipes, used throughout this book provide healthy alternatives to more common, similar preparations.

YOGURT CHEESE

Use this light and creamy cheese as a substitute for cream cheese. To create a cheese with the consistency of cream cheese, place a plate directly on top of the draining yogurt and refrigerate for 8 hours. Store in a tightly covered container in the refrigerator for up to 5 days.

Makes 1 cup (8 oz/250 g)

2 cups (16 oz/500 g) lowfat plain yogurt
2 tablespoons fresh orange juice
grated zest of ½ orange
1½ tablespoons honey

1. Spoon the yogurt into a coffee cone fitted with a paper filter. Place the cone over a bowl and let drain at room temperature for at least 8 hours or overnight. Discard the whey or use it for another purpose. The longer the yogurt drains, the thicker the cheese will be.
2. Transfer to a bowl or other container and stir in the orange juice, zest and honey. Cover tightly and chill well before using.

Per 1 Tablespoon Serving: Calories 20 (Kilojoules 83), Protein 1 g, Carbohydrates 3 g, Total Fat 0 g, Saturated Fat 0 g, Cholesterol 1 mg, Sodium 9 mg, Dietary Fiber 0 g

RICOTTA ICING

Although there is no butter in this delicious lowfat icing, it has a buttery quality that makes it wonderful for spreading on cakes or cookies. It takes less than 20 minutes to make and can be stored in a tightly covered container in the refrigerator for up to 1 week. Do not attempt to freeze the icing, however, as it separates when frozen.

Makes 1 cup (8 fl oz/250 ml)

¾ cup (6 oz/185 g) lowfat ricotta cheese
¼ cup (2 oz/60 g) lowfat plain yogurt
¼ teaspoon vanilla extract (essence)
¼ teaspoon almond extract (essence)
¹⁄₁₆ teaspoon freshly grated nutmeg

1. In a food processor fitted with the metal blade, combine the ricotta cheese, yogurt, vanilla and almond extracts and nutmeg and process until well combined, about 30 seconds.
2. Cover and chill for 15 minutes before using.

Per 1 Tablespoon Serving: Calories 16 (Kilojoules 67), Protein 2 g, Carbohydrates 1 g, Total Fat 1 g, Saturated Fat 0 g, Cholesterol 2 mg, Sodium 16 mg, Dietary Fiber 0 g

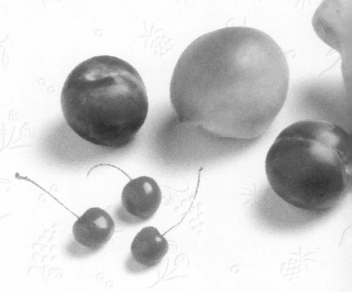

VANILLA SUGAR

Sugar in which a vanilla bean has been buried adds a deep vanilla flavor to anything in which the sugar is used. A vanilla bean that has already been used in cooking can be used once again to make vanilla sugar. Be sure the vanilla bean is thoroughly dry before adding it to the sugar. Store in a tightly covered container at room temperature for 6 months.

Makes 4 cups (2 lb/1 kg)

4 cups (2 lb/1 kg) granulated or confectioners'
  (icing) sugar
1 vanilla bean

1. In a bowl, combine the sugar and vanilla bean. Store in a tightly covered container. It will be ready to use in 3 days.

Per 1 Tablespoon Serving: Calories 55 (Kilojoules 232), Protein 0 g, Carbohydrates 14 g, Total Fat 0 g, Saturated Fat 0 g, Cholesterol 0 mg, Sodium 0 mg, Dietary Fiber 0 g

FRUIT COULIS

Raspberries are the most commonly used fruits for making a fruit coulis, or sauce, but almost any fruit can be used: blackberries, blueberries, cherries, kiwifruits, passion fruits, peaches, nectarines, mangoes or drained canned crushed pineapple. Adjust the amount of sugar depending upon the sweetness of the fruit.

Makes about 1 cup (8 fl oz/250 ml)

2 cups (8 oz/250 g) stemmed berries or
  diced, peeled and pitted fruit or 1 package
  (12 oz/375 g) frozen berries, thawed,
  including juice
1 tablespoon fresh lemon juice
3 tablespoons superfine (caster) sugar

1. In a food processor fitted with the metal blade, purée the berries or other fruit until smooth. Alternatively, place the berries or fruit in a bowl and crush with a potato masher. If you have used raspberries or other berries with seeds and want to remove the seeds, pass the sauce through a sieve into a bowl.
2. Mix in the lemon juice and sugar and serve, or cover and refrigerate for up to 3 days.

Per 1 Tablespoon Serving: Calories 16 (Kilojoules 68), Protein 0 g, Carbohydrates 4 g, Total Fat 0 g, Saturated Fat 0 g, Cholesterol 0 mg, Sodium 0 mg, Dietary Fiber 1 g

LOWFAT PASTRY

A flour that is low in protein, and thus low in gluten when mixed with liquid, helps to produce a tender crust. The use of a low-protein cake flour is especially important when the fat level is as low as it is in this pastry. Lowfat cream cheese adds richness to the pastry, with less fat than an equivalent amount of butter would add.

Makes one 9-inch (23-cm) pie or tart crust

1½ cups (6 oz/185 g) cake (soft-wheat) flour
¹⁄₁₆ teaspoon sea salt
2 tablespoons vegetable shortening or unsalted
   butter, chilled, thinly sliced
3 tablespoons lowfat cream cheese, chilled, cut
   into small dice
6 tablespoons (3 fl oz/90 ml) cold water

1. In a mixing bowl, combine the flour and salt and stir to blend. Add the shortening or butter and cream cheese and, using your fingers (which must be very cold) or a pastry blender, work the ingredients together until the mixture is the texture of coarse meal.

2. Using a fork, stir in the water, 1 or 2 tablespoons at a time, and toss the flour mixture to form a ball. Alternatively, place the flour and salt in the work bowl of a food processor fitted with the metal blade. Pulse once to combine. Add the shortening and cream cheese. Pulse several times until the mixture forms dough the size of small peas. Add the cold water. Pulse 3 or 4 times, just until the dough starts to form a ball and leave the sides of the bowl. Do not overmix or the pastry will be tough.

3. Wrap in waxed paper and refrigerate for 5–30 minutes, to make sure it is cold once again.

4. To use, on a lightly floured work surface, roll out the dough into an 11-inch (28-cm) round for a pie pan or a 10-inch (25-cm) round for a tart pan with a removable bottom. Drape the round over the rolling pin and transfer it to a 9-inch (23-cm) pie pan or tart pan. Gently ease the dough into the pan. If using a pie pan, trim the overhang to ½ inch (12 mm). Fold the overhang under and crimp the edge. If using a tart pan, cut off the pastry even with the rim.

Per Crust: Calories 1,086 (Kilojoules 4,562), Protein 22 g, Carbohydrates 169 g, Total Fat 35 g, Saturated Fat 11 g, Cholesterol 22 mg, Sodium 332 mg, Dietary Fiber 0 g

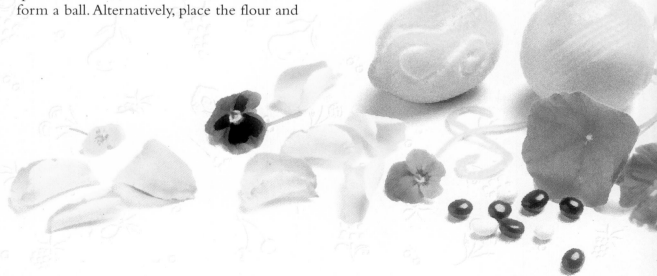

LOWFAT CRÈME ANGLAISE

The addition of cornstarch reduces the number of eggs needed to make this traditional custard sauce, thus dramatically reducing the fat. Use this Crème Anglaise as a sauce over cakes and cobblers or as a base for ice cream. To thicken the Crème Anglaise to use for a pie filling, increase the cornstarch to ¼ cup (1 oz/30 g). Store in the refrigerator for up to 1 week.

Makes about 2 cups (16 fl oz/500 ml)

2 cups (16 fl oz/500 ml) lowfat milk
¼ cup (2 oz/60 g) sugar
3 tablespoons cornstarch (cornflour)
1 egg yolk
2 teaspoons vanilla extract (essence)

1. In a small saucepan over medium heat, warm the milk until small bubbles form along the edges of the pan. At the same time, in a separate saucepan, combine the sugar and cornstarch.

2. Gradually stir the hot milk into the sugar mixture, mixing until blended. Place over medium heat and cook, stirring constantly, until the mixture thickens, about 5 minutes.

3. In a small bowl, whisk the egg yolk until lightly beaten. Whisk a few tablespoons of the hot milk mixture into the egg yolk, then whisk the yolk mixture into the saucepan. Cook over low heat, stirring constantly, until the mixture thickens enough to coat the back of a spoon, about 5 minutes. Run your finger through the custard on the spoon; if the line remains, the custard is ready. Do not allow the custard to come to a boil or it will curdle. Stir in the vanilla extract.

4. Pour the mixture into a bowl. Cover with plastic wrap to prevent a skin from forming and let cool. Use the sauce immediately or refrigerate.

Per 1 Tablespoon Serving: Calories 19 (Kilojoules 81), Protein 1 g, Carbohydrates 3 g, Total Fat 0 g, Saturated Fat 0 g, Cholesterol 8 mg, Sodium 8 mg, Dietary Fiber 0 g

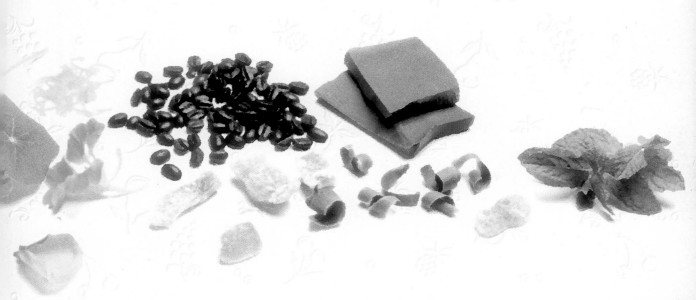

INDEX